Magic Mushrooms

The Definitive Step-by-step Guide to Cultivation

(A Simple Guide to Home Cultivation of Psychedelic Mushrooms)

Melissa Dubois

Published By **Regina Ioviusher**

Melissa Dubois

All Rights Reserved

Magic Mushrooms: The Definitive Step-by-step Guide to Cultivation (A Simple Guide to Home Cultivation of Psychedelic Mushrooms)

ISBN   978-1-77485-474-7

No part of this guidebook shall be reproduced in any form without permission in writing from the publisher except in the case of brief quotations embodied in critical articles or reviews.

Legal & Disclaimer

The information contained in this ebook is not designed to replace or take the place of any form of medicine or professional medical advice. The information in this ebook has been provided for educational & entertainment purposes only.

The information contained in this book has been compiled from sources deemed reliable, and it is accurate to the best of the Author's knowledge; however, the Author cannot guarantee its accuracy and validity and cannot be held liable for any errors or omissions. Changes are periodically made to this book. You must consult your doctor or get professional medical advice before using any of the suggested remedies, techniques, or information in this book.

TABLE OF CONTENTS

Introduction

Mind-altering substances like mushrooms, has been observed throughout the history of humanity regardless of whether they are used for aiding rituals of worship to experience "spiritual conscious" or for recreational use. These substances, sometimes known as drugs are now a part of our society.

Their use has been criticized by many and this criticism within the legal community is the reason for their abolition across the world, mainly because of the findings of research conducted by scientists that claim they harm the human body as well as the psyche. The consumption of these mushrooms is prohibited due to social guidelines.

However, it's the results of scientific research that have been the catalyst for the continued existence of the debate on "to take or not" since research has demonstrated how these "drugs" have a positive impact on the health of human beings.

The mushrooms which are part of the legal discussion aren't ones that can help create delicious risotto that tastes great or those that we normally find on pizzas. Nor are they the kinds that are poisonous or toxic and could cause death. The mushrooms considered beneficial and damaging while at the same time are those that belong to the psychedelic type. They are also known by the name of "magic mushroom." What is different about them from other kinds of mushrooms is the chemical "psilocybin," which produces hallucinogenic effects for the users.

If you'd like to participate in this kind of experience, how are you going to ensure you can determine which one is safe and gives you the desired outcomes? You might even be wondering the dangers or value of the drugs could be for you.

This guide aims to give the answers to queries like these and many more. As a guide to magical mushrooms, it will give information about the background of their use, as well as details on the various kinds and which ones are the most beneficial to consume.

It will also guide you in identifying these mushrooms, assisting you to discern between psilocybin-producing mushrooms and those that can cause fatal.

Additionally, you will be able to learn more about the numerous studies that provide information about the ways that magic mushrooms can help improve your health, as well as research on mental illnesses, cancer and various ailments.

If your curiosity has been so keen and you want to grow the mushrooms for personal usage this guide will provide you the necessary steps to cultivate them in your own backyard.

The information that is objective throughout this guide will provide an insight at the various positive and negative side effects of these substances. It is our hope that, at the end of this book this book, you will be able to better understand the magic mushrooms and will be able to create your own conclusion

about the reasons for using the psychoactive
mushrooms.

Chapter 1: What Magic Musshrooms?

Magic mushrooms, in the way they're known are fungi that occur naturally that are usually consumed fresh or dried and can be consumed as tea or coffee. They can cause hallucinogenic effects in the person who consumes them.

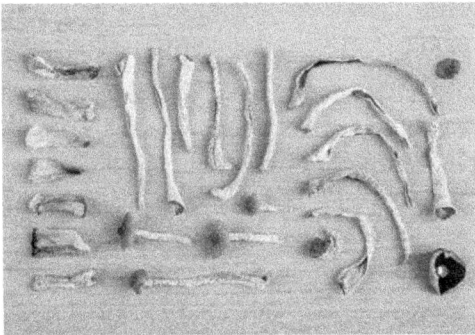

Dried Magic Mushrooms

There are a variety of magic mushrooms that offer varying levels in hallucinogenic properties. In the end, preparation techniques and the method of consumption depend on the individual user. If the consumption results in gratifying results or even a terrifying experience, it isn't something that the user can control. It usually takes less than an hour for the point of your "trip" in order to experience hallucinations or experiencing hallucinations, and these effects can last as long as 6 hours per day. It's comparable (and is a less drastic option) to the more hazardous chemical hallucinogen, semi-synthetically known as LSD.

Magic mushrooms are typically made by massaging, and then consumed when mixed into drinks or food however, some people consume fresh harvested magic mushrooms.

They also are known by "street name.," such as:

* Shrooms,

* Mushies,

* Blue meanies,

* Gold shirts

* Freedom caps

* Philosopher's stones,

* Liberties,

* Amani,

* Easy simon,

* Smokey cigarette,

* Cubes,

* Fire in the color of purple,

Holy mushrooms!

* Smokey cigarette,

* Zoomers,

* Boomers,

* And Agaric.

The long-term consequences of taking magic mushrooms could cause poisoning, the biggest obstacle to reducing this is the normal availability (they are more prevalent in grazing areas that are wild or around cow and horse stool).

This could be a bit of a naivete to those who are enthralled by mushrooms who go out to collect themselves in the belief that each mushroom is edible.

But not all of these parasites are the most desirable ones and it's difficult to identify which are harmful or not. Certain of them have proven to be extremely poisonous, and may kill you in a very painful and slow manner that can cause symptoms such as nausea diarrhoea, fever, and nausea.

Some suffer from a delayed reaction that takes a while to display symptoms or signs before committing suicide. There is no cure to treat this kind of reaction.

Poisonous Mushrooms

Because magic mushrooms naturally occurring, and not synthesized prior to consumption They're often viewed as a safe treatment.

There is no guarantee that a medication is safe as many drugs are created or manufactured by organic plants and fungi. However they're not an addictive or heavy-dosed medication.

They're not as emotional or violent like LSD or crack, and they aren't not corroding in the same way as crack or heroin. Based on the user's mental state, they could affect the user.

For instance, if the person is more susceptible to developing a mental state or is clearly an extremely impressionable person They might believe that their hallucinations may be a sign of something genuine and get a bit obsessed with it and eventually be damaged by it.

These documented examples of extremes include one where the child began taking mushrooms, and was able to have constant hallucinations of a flower dressed as a court-jester , who made fun of him by hurling insults.

As bizarre as it may sound and without even denying these hallucinations, he was convinced that this flower was a sign of his own misperceptions about himself. it led him to depression that was severe.

His friends and he believed that he was perfectly good before taking the mushrooms. However, somewhere in the course of time, the adverse effects began to show.

Unfortunately, even to the present, he battles with psychological and emotional problems that weren't present prior to the life-altering hallucinations caused through the mushrooms.

It is impossible to be certain in this instance whether or not the mushrooms played a role in causing these ongoing mental problems or if it was an intrinsic mental illness was caused by the mushroom is important to keep in mind.

In the past, it was believed that it was the reckless hippies and teens who were able to take part in magical mushrooms, but it's not so. According to two researches conducted recently magical mushrooms, and maybe even the medicine psilocybin could have significant benefits for cancer patients who suffer with depression and stress.

Just one (1) dose provided the majority of patients relief from their stress within six months. Many were stress-free for years afterward.

A Group of Psilocybin Mushrooms

According to studies the magical mushrooms helped ease anxiety and depression because of the feeling as "you". This causes a change within the mind, also known as neuroplasticity.

Studies using MRI imaging have shown that psilocybin affects brain activity which allows for communication between brain regions which typically don't connect.

In a newspaper article on December 1st, 2016 an Time Magazine article, Dinah Bazer recounts her experience by taking a single dose of psilocybin as part of her study at NYU Langone Medical Centre.

Dinah said that initially, she felt fear and felt as if she was "glancing across the universe." After being guided by researchers, she was able to unravel and see her dread as a dark mass in her body. She took over and moved the black mass outside and it went away.

She "... started to experience love-like. I felt like my body was kissed by love , and it was amazing, gorgeous, beautiful... The sensation of love that was so overwhelming continued for months, and even four decades later, I sometimes feel as if I'm experiencing it. My anxiety and fear was completely eliminated and have never returned... This experience altered the way I'd like to live my existence... I'd like to imagine what it would be like if the cancer returned, but I'm not thinking about it the same way.

Although I don't feel well, and thoughts of return of the same thing creep into my mind I lack dread and simply belie. Let's just wait and observe the outcome."

Whatever is going on must come Down

While the benefits of magic mushrooms appear promising, according to Stephen Ross, who headed the NYU study, "If somebody goes out and does it by themselves be a victim, they may feel extreme anxiety and fear and experience a greater sense of anxiety. Although I'm sympathetic however, I strongly advise people not to do this."

Even in controlled environments We are uncertain that the benefits of mushrooms that are magical outweigh dangers. It is a reminder of how people are now claiming that marijuana bongs have very little or no side negative effects. Similar to how we didn't have to be thinking about it until the age of our late teens, now we have come to believe that all drugs can affect the psychological and emotional well-being, hinder religious development and could entice bad items and demons of religion.

It is also important to be aware of the physiological effects of swallowing mind-altering medications (and additional alcohol) and alcohol, which could result in deficiency in vitamins and minerals, liver issues as well as cognitive problems and many more.

THE ENTIRE HISTORY CONCISE OF MUSSHROOMS

Many historians believe that magic mushrooms were used as a source of energy in 9000 B.C. within North African indigenous civilizations, according to the representations found of stone artworks discovered throughout Spain as well as Algeria. Statues as well as other representations of what appear to be mushrooms were also found inside Aztec and Mayan ruin sites located in Central America. The Aztecs employed a material called teonanacatl, which translates as "flesh of the gods" which many believe was magic mushrooms.

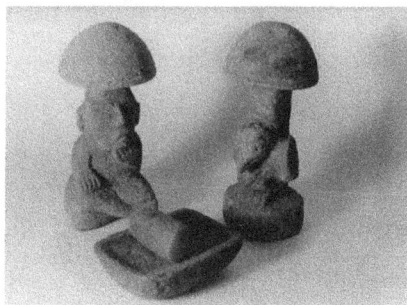

Maya Mushroom Stones

Alongside peyote, dawn glory seeds, and other psychotropics that naturally occur, these substances have been used to create a trance that creates visions and talk to gods. Following the time that Spanish Catholic missionary priests arrived in the New World from the 16th century, many of them wrote about the use of these substances.

14

The idea of magical mushrooms having a long and sacred history is highly controversial. Many believe that no evidence is definitive, and that people see exactly what they'd like to see in the earliest artworks, sculptures and manuscripts. There is however, evidence of support for use within a variety of modern tribes of indigenous peoples from Central America, such as the Mazatec, Mixtec, Nauhua and Zapatec.

Magic mushrooms began to be consumed by Westerners during the 1950s. A mycologist (one who investigates mushroom research), R. Gordon Wasson traveled across Mexico to study mushrooms in the year 1955. He participated and observed an ancient ritual that used magical mushrooms. It was led by a shaman from the Mazatec native people and women from the Oaxaca region in southern Mexico. Wasson published his findings in a journal that was published inside Life magazine in 1957. The title was conceived by an editor "Seeking the magic mushroom" and a guide on the genesis of the term, but Wasson did not use the term. Some of his coworkers, Roger Heim had enjoyed the help

15

from Albert Hofmann (the "father" of LSD) and he was able to isolate and extract psilocybin and Psilocin from the mushrooms Heim along with Wasson brought back from Mexico. This is the reason he decided to establish The Harvard Psilcybin Project.

Dr. Timoty Leary

Timothy Leary, possibly the most well-known advocate of psychotropic medicines such as LSD The author read the Life article. It has piqued his curiosity. He founded the Harvard Psilocybin Project to study its effects on the substance on individuals. From then on, the magical mushrooms became a part of the fabric to the hippie movement , along with their own search for new spirituality forms and spirituality for the rest of the decade.

The 1970s brought the prohibition of psilocybin only in clinical research. These have only recently reopened after more than 30 years.

Who would have thought that certain kinds of mushrooms have amazing health benefits? The research carried out by Associate Professor Min

Zhang, School of Population Health at the University of Western Australia, on the beneficial effects of ingestion of the mushrooms of girls China proves that the Agaricus family of mushrooms have an unique power that is often unnoticed and can help us become healthier.

THE RETURN OF THE MAGIC MUSHROOM

Super Mario fans Super Mario may notice mushrooms in the game. Research scientists are conducting more studies on the mushrooms, as well as chefs from all over the globe cook using mushrooms. They appear overnight and disappear in a flash, and do not leave any trace of the experience.

The people who study the fungus are called mycologists. Today the fungus is thought of as a possible cure for obesity, cancer, PTSD (Post-traumatic Stress Disorder) and other mental disorders.

Mushrooms Laboratory Analysis

Mushrooms, sometimes referred to as toadstools, are a type of fungi that are found over the soil or in an edible resource. They are distinct from the world of plants in a kingdom known as Myceteae because they don't contain chlorophyll like plants.

In the absence of the photosynthesis process some mushrooms get nutrition through the breakdown of organic matter, or by taking in higher plant material. They are referred to as decomposers. A different kind of decomposer eats living plants in order to kill and consume them. They're also known as parasites.

Tree Mushrooms

Forms that are poisonous and edible are mycorrhizal and are found close to or on the branches of trees such as pines, oaks and firs.

For people, mushrooms could serve as a remedy for the three (3) things namely nourishment, cure or poison. Some are harmless. The three most popular edible varieties from the "meat of the world of vegetables'" would be the oyster, the morel and the chanterelles.

They're widely used in cooking throughout China, Korea, Japan and India. In reality, China is the world's largest producer, accounting for over half of all mushrooms consumed worldwide.

The vast majority of the food variety we find in our grocery stores are produced commercially using trucks, and include varieties like the portobello, shiitake, and enoki.

Shiitake Mushrooms

Portobello Mushrooms

Enoki Mushrooms

Eastern medicine, specifically the traditional Chinese clinics, have employed mushrooms for many years. In the U.S., research was initiated in the early 60s in search of methods that could manage the immune system, as well as to stop tumour growth by using extracts in research on cancer.

Over the course of the century that has followed, more than 40,000 patients were awarded psilocybin as well as other hallucinogens such as LSD as well as mescaline. More than 1,000 research papers were written. After the authorities became aware of the growing subculture that was willing to embrace the use of mushrooms, rules were introduced.

In 1970, the Nixon Administration started rules, which formed the Controlled Substances Act of 1970. The law established five programs of increasing severity that required medication to be classified. Psilocybin was categorized as the most restrictive, along alongside marijuana as well as MDMA. Each was described as having an "high possibility of abuse, no current accepted medical use, and a deficiency of security standards that are accepted."

The study was stopped for nearly 25 years until recent research began the possibility of possible applications in dealing with or resolving PTSD disorder in conjunction with stress related issues. The study was conducted in June of 2014. complete extracts or mushrooms were examined within 32 research trials conducted by the U.S. National Institutes of Health due to their potential effects on a variety of diseases and conditions. Certain illnesses that are that are being treated include cancer, immunity and pneumonia, as well as inflammatory bowel disease.

The topic of controversy is the use of psilocybin, which is an organic compound found in certain types of mushrooms. Its ability to help those suffering from psychological disorders such as obsessive compulsive disorder stress, and PTSD is still being studied. Psilocybin is also proven as more efficient at combating addiction to cigarettes cigarettes and smoking cigarettes in specific studies.

Mushrooms Laboratory Analysis

Although the fungi have been a fascination for people for a long time, they are now entering an age of new discovery, with their healing abilities and unexplored properties have been discovered. The fungus may be the answer to a long line of mystery as well as illnesses.

Mycology, the study of mushrooms is drawing new researchers that want to investigate the "fungus in the lives of people." The fungus is used for a range of health-related reasons all over all over the world, the humble toadstool may be able to come into the spotlight in a matter of minutes and as an effective alternative solution to a number of stubborn pains.

The popularity of mushrooms among growers is due to their rich nutrients. For instance, they make vitamin D in the presence of the sun. Mushrooms are rich in B-vitamins, Vitamin C potassium, calcium, phosphorus and calcium. They also contain sodium, calcium and zinc.

Medicinal mushrooms have tens of tens of thousands of nutrients and compounds which are health-strengthening. Eastern medicine, specifically conventional Chinese clinics, has relied on mushrooms for a long time. Within the U.S., research have been conducted since the beginning of the 60s on possible methods to control the immune system as well as to prevent the development of cancerous tumours by using the extracts of fungi.

Mushroom hunting is a favored activity across the world However, it's not always secure. A lot of edible mushrooms are identical to poisonous ones. It's up to a specialist to determine the distinction. Furthermore, they act like sponges and absorb the toxins of the environment and dirt. However, they can be easily considered "healthy."

The medicinal use of mushrooms is taking place now in the past few centuries, and with good reasons - they're highly effective. It's the time to conduct more thorough studies into the other uses and potential of this delicate gifts of nature.

Magic mushrooms have been found in the wild or cultivated, that contain Psilocybin, a natural psychoactive that is associated with hallucinogenic chemicals. Psilocybin is considered to be among the most popular psychedelics in accordance with the Substance Addiction and Mental Health Service Administration's. Psilocybin is classified as an Schedule I drug, meaning it has a significant potential for abuse and does not have any currently recognized medical therapy within the USA.

KINDS OF MUSHROOMS THAT MAGIC

The process of hunting for wild mushrooms can be dangerous. There are also hundreds of species, which means there are many that have similar abilities. Some poisonous mushrooms could cause stomach problems however, others can result in organ failure and even death. Finding any kind of wild mushroom is recommended for those who have a solid understanding of the identification of mushrooms. Even those who have been looking for the wild for a long time have made mistakes. One of the components of this identification technique is the creation of print based on spores, which involves pressing the cap's gill side down on a piece of newspaper (typically both black and white for a comparison) which is how spores are printed. (We will go into more detail about the potential applications of printing spores later.)

There are numerous species of animals belonging to the Genus psilocybe. Most of them are on the opposite side of the spectrum - the typical size is 3 inches tall as well as a 1-inch cap. As they grow, they typically have yellow, light greyish or brown stems, with caps of brownish or brown with white and dark gills.

There are over 100 kinds of magical mushrooms, but the most popular ones are believed to be:

* Psilocybe azurescens (greatest psilocybin material)

* Psilocybe bohemica (next greatest psilocybin material)

* Conocbe Cyanopus

* Copelandia cyanescens

* Panaeolus africanus

* Panaeolus subbalteus

* Inocybe aeruginascens

* Psilocybe cubensis

* Psilocybe Cyescens

* Psilocybe mexicana

* Psilocybe semilanceata

* Psilocybe tampanensis

Let's examine several of the popular varieties in greater detail.

Psilocybe cubensis

Psilocybe cubensis can be found on the higher end as it is magical mushrooms are involved. It is also one of the most commonly encountered. It is referred to as the common large psilocybe, gold Mexican or cap mulch. It comes in a variety of different varieties. The cover is usually red-brown, and has the stem being yellow or white. When crushed or crushed its fleshy, tacky is able to be seen.

Psilocybe cubensis

Many believe that this is an absolute sign of the presence of the magical mushroom, but certain poisonous types of mushrooms can also cause bruises. They are usually found in humid and damp climates. It also grows from the dung of cattle and other animals that are grazing, like.

Psilocybe semilanceata

Psilocybe semilanceata also known as freedom cap is a common psilocybin fungus. Generally, P. semilanceata. It can be found in areas of mountainous and moist soil typically frequented by cows.

Psilocybe semilanceata

Although it is similar to P. cubensis, this is not able to grow in the soil. It's a small mushroom, which is either bright yellow or brown, with caps that are rather pointed. The other psilocybe species, Psilocybe pelliculosa, is often mistaken for P. semilanceata. However its characteristics are a bit less.

Psilocybe baeocystis

Psilocybe baeocystis has an dark brown cover as well as the stem is yellow or brown when it is reenergizing.

Psilocybe baeocystis

It is often seen in the vicinity as well as it growing on rotting logs such as peat or compost. Nicknames include the powerful Psilocybeblue bell and the cap of a jar.

IDENTIFYING MUSSHROOMS

The identification of wild mushrooms can be a daunting task and must be handled with care. By studying this guide, you're likely identify the most basic features which are essential to identify the species of mushrooms. You can use this guide to make the list of things to record and check in the event of encountering an unknown species. The recognition of mushrooms is also an enjoyable pastime to enhance your hikes with friends, and with the right information, it makes it possible to hunt for the best edibles you can come across. This isn't a replace a thorough study of the region and a thorough knowledge of mosquito colonies.

1. Examining Time and Place

A. Find out what food items you'd think of finding to your location and the time of day.

B. Find out what kinds of mushrooms are located in your region of the world. This will reduce your options of species that could be possible.

C. Note the date. Some mushrooms are only situated in a particular interval (spring/summer/fall/winter).

2. Look for the fungus that grows on

A. Organic product:

In the form of foliage

Compost

O Soil

B. On wood:

Live on sterile timber

o Softwood or Hardwood

Species of tree

3. Determine the species and the level of safety once the mushroom is identified as a part of any of the species of trees. This could mean that it is an mycorrhizal, or perhaps parasitic bacteria. Mycorrhizal fungi typically occur in the root systems of trees. They are located around the trees' foundations as well as extending out. This can be difficult to recognize, particularly when the number of species decreases.

It is Mycorrhizal fungi are more prevalent when a normal radial form the base of the shrub.

O Mycorrhizal fungi can form Tethered fairy circles at the top of live as well dead tree.

The Parasitic Fungi may grow at the bottom of the tree, directly or in the wood.

Also, be aware of your place and what kinds of mushrooms can be enlarged. Additionally, take note that fungal networks can persist even after a tree has died.

4. Note your surroundings. Certain species require specific surroundings for growth.

o Meadow

o Wetlands/floodplains

Moist or dry area of forests

What kind of forest you're in (deciduous or coniferous or mixed)

O Sandy or dry conditions

O Coastal regions

5. Analyzing whether the Pileus or Cap

A. Check the type of cap. Also, take note of the age in the live mushroom. Does it look:

Convex - A smooth dome-shaped cap.

Ovoid or Hemispherical - Just like half of an egg.

O Campanulate - Bell-shaped.

Conical - Cone-like appearance.

O Umbonate - Featuring an umbo basic (a curving and bulge) as well as a cap that is flat.

O Umbilicate - With an ordinary round depression similar to umbonate's reverse.

O Papillate - With an oblique bulge in the middle of pay.

Funnel - Steep sadness centrally, creating an funnel.

Sunken - Cap grey with margins greater than the central.

o Flat - A planar cap.

O Cylindrical - A rounded shirt that has an extremely large Perpendicular Cap (e.g. shaggy hair).

O Bracket - Shelf-like limitations climbing on wood; generally in the form of a fan.

Spherical - Completely around; only found in volva puffballs and unbroken.

B. Look at the cross-sectional margin of the cap. Examine the manner in which the surface of the cap meet. Do you think it's:

Straight - The end of the cap on the same plane, there is no curve.

o Incurved/Downturned – The pay arch's edge down.

Recurved/Upturned - The end of cap arch towards the upwards.

Involute - Edge the pay that is curled down.

Revolute - Finalization of cap curled upward.

Rounded - The edge of the pay-around.

Sterile - When that the cap's edge extends past the surface of the spore.

C. Examine the summary of the perimeter. Are you able to:

o Entire/Smooth - Unbroken outline.

O Scalloped - Has regularity of semicircles.

o Striate - Short, parallel ridges.

The olbed's margins cleave into the inside, similar to the lobes on a plant.

O Sinuate Swirly borders.

O Cracked/Rimose - Splits within the cap's along the perimeter.

Appendiculate - Collectively, with veins turning off the perimeter.

D. Check the texture and appearance that the cap has. Does it look:

Smooth To the Touch.

Velvety - Hairs that are tiny which are fragile when touched to the bottom.

Scales - Close overlapped fibres on the cap like scales.

O Corrugated - Wrinkled in appearance and texture.

O Hairy - Fibrous could be a bit shaggy.

o Areolate - A busted routine, quite like paint.

Warts - Remains from an old veil that smudges over the upper layer.

Viscid - Dry and slimy (often can be seen in the middle).

O Waxy Cap - Cap coated with an outer coat that is smooth.

O Zonate – Concentric groups of color (e.g. the turkey tail).

6. Look for the features of the hymenium the surface of the spore.

A. Examine the bottom of your specimen, and then locate the surface of the spore. Take note of the appearance of the spore. The most commonly used varieties are:

O Lamellae - Gills that cover the floor, relatively small and fragile.

Pores - A decorative coating that is surrounded by tubes, that could be regarded as holes.

Teeth - Icicle-like structures that hang down.

or False Gills - Fleecy ridges that surround the hymenium. They could look to be Gills (e.g. or an chanterelle).

O Gleba - The spore-producing interior Puffballs' flesh.

B. Find the place where the gills join the Stem and look at the patterns of attachment. Are they:

O Free - Gills don't reach the to the stem.

Gills can be attached only when the base and stem match.

Adnate - Attached to the stem to provide a complete diameter for the gill (right).

O Decurrent - Gills move across stem cells.

The Collarium Gills do not extend to the stem, but are connected to an elongated collar.

Sinuate - Top of the line in the gills, before moving through the stem.

C. Examine the gills to check if they're spread out beneath the cap. Are they:

Gills in the extreme distance.

o Close Gills - Close together but using described spacing between.

Gills spells out quite.

The space is huge between the Gills.

7. Examining your Stipe or Stem

A. Find out the status of the stem. Check the bottom of the clog at the point where the stem and the clog meet. Do you see:

Central - It is located in the middle of pay.

O Exocentric - Offset to the center in the cap.

O Lateral - Stem that is to be in accordance with the entire caps (not the vertical).

O Sessile - Stem is not present.

B. Find out the type of stem. Take note of the base which might be covered or underground. Does it look like:

Equal - Equal length across the stem.

O Clavate o Clavate Stem grows in size as it approaches the base, for example, an oath.

O Bulbous - Base of stem cells that are often covered, is believed like an onion.

The Volva is a cup-like sac that is located at the stem's base (remains of the global veil).

O Tapered - Stem becomes more scaly near the bottom.

Radicating - A stem that has a slim, root-like arrangement at the base.

C. Take a look from the perspective as well as the appearance. Consider the colour as well as other features of the surface. Stem texture is typically important in Boletes (stem cells) and helps shield hens with pores).

Smooth - Soft to the touch.

O Scabers - Small scaber like fibres that run through the stem. Pay attention to the color.

or Glandular Dots - Dots that are colored around the stem. They are also an unremarkable feature to identify Suillus mushrooms.

or Scales - A warty or darker layout.

Reticulate--A net-like design or weathered look of the stem.

D. Check the inside. Utilizing a sharp knife, make an incision along the stem's base and the cap if required and the goal is to examine the cross-section that the mushroom has. Are you able to tell:

O Powerful - A absorption.

Tubular - Hollow tube running through center.

Hollow-Lean partitions.

O Fibrous - A thread-like inside.

E. Find the tight veil at the purpose that is present. The surface of the spores is covered when it is young, and matures at maturity, leaving indications. This isn't a characteristic in many species of mushrooms. Examine the stem to find any vestiges of a veil. remains may take on different forms like:

Sheath - Extensions of the outer coat of stalks and sticks like vase.

Twist Zone A ring, or mark made from the thin veil.

O Flaring - Stiff ring can be seen outside.

o Pendant - Skirt-like ring.

o Cortinate - Cobweb-like fibres.

O Slimy - Many mushrooms have a coating of slime, which forms a veil.

8. Thinking about patterns of growth and Spores

A. Analyze the entire design of this specimen and also the locations for other specimens. Look for patterns at the location the place they begin to develop. The most common designs include:

O Cespitose is a plant that grows from clusters of compacted clumps and stems packed or fused with each other (e.g., Enoki).

O Gregarious - Growing in separate but with tiny clusters.

O Solitary - Always seen alone or invisible within an area.

A Fairy Ring growing radially out in areas around tree.

O Imbricate - Shelf-like expanding sides of wood within close proximity and often overlapped.

B. Use a spore print. If the spores are not visible in or around the mushroom it is best to seek out an spore printing in order to find the color. For deciding on a print you'll need an adroit knife as well as paper and containers. If you've taken the proper steps to take an image, it will be easy to discern the colour of spores that are left.

o Make sure the mulch is old enough to allow spores to be deposited in contrast to being overly old.

Make use of a sterilized knife to separate the cap and stem as quickly as you're in a position to.

Place the cap on top and then place it spore-side-down on your own piece of paper.

Cover the paper with an airtight container to restrict the flow of air. Allow the specimen to sit on in the paper for a few hours.

Once the mulch has dried, either inside or outside and you are ready to remove a wet napkin inside the cap. Make sure not to dampen the paper, or the spores could be difficult to spot.

9. Fragrant Distinct Characteristics

A. Examine to determine whether the lumps of flesh are particular colours. Certain mushrooms might be able to lighten blue or other colors when the flesh inside gets exposed to oxygen. This can be a distinctive characteristic of some species of fungi. To determine busing potential:

Ensure that the mushroom is old enough to allow for a test.

o Locate an unexplored area inside your specimen's stem cap.

The mushroom can be cool, it is possible to make one tiny cut or an emotional ache using your fingers.

Watch the mark you've created. If it doesn't break within 10 to 15 minutes, it's most likely to not be damaged by any color.

Examine the color of the bruising. The colour blue is most popular colour however certain species may blossom in red or black.

B. Look for any forms of latex created by this particular mushroom. Some mushrooms are able to leak a sterile chemical referred to as latex. The entire lactarius genus has this characteristic. They're often called wheat caps. The latex can be a variety of distinct colors and could react to your skin or air changing colours. To determine if a mushroom produces this substance:

o Ensure the mushroom is clean enough to produce latex. Typically, old specimens are likely to dry out.

Utilize a knife to make a small cut, at the point at the point where the gills and the stem can be found or the gills are positioned to can be inserted into the cap.

Watch for the any ooze of latex. If it doeshappen, observe it every 3 to 5 minutes. Watch for any changes in colour. You should wait for 1 or 2 hours to determine whether there was a reaction.

You should learn about the skin and latex color, since a crucial feature could be the colour reaction between the two. As an example an example, a mushroom that has skin and latex that is white could eventually be stained purple due to the particular contact.

C. Note any distinct smells.

Although it isn't a major characteristic for many mushrooms smell could be an important characteristic. Examine the mushrooms and observe if the smell has a distinct smell or is "off." Cut off several stems or caps when the smell is less.

Mushrooms that KILL

The fascinating world of fungus is endless and there are a variety of varieties. It is a species of plant that do not produce chlorophyll and, therefore, don't require sunlight to grow. They have plenty of space to develop and flourish, which is worthwhile researching. One of the most sought-after varieties is the ones we consume.

The yeast, for instance, is a parasite that people utilize in cooking, as well as mushrooms. They can be very delicious and it is possible to become addicted to them. This is the reason they may be quite expensive to purchase.

Some species are toxic and can be carried and transmitted by insects, animals and many other species. Fungi that are transported via of a frog for example, was brought into the Americas from the 1930s to the 1950s. It was utilized to detect if women were pregnant.

The mushroom was released into the wild, and the result is that there is a global loss of many species of frogs, and perhaps even salamanders. This alone shows that the addition of species from one continent to another often leads to devastating consequences for the fauna of the region. The Cane Toad, which was introduced to Australia around the same time caused a massive impact on the local wildlife because of the poison it dispenses.

Mouldsand smuts and rusts, as well as yeast as well as mould falls are part of the category of fungi. Although we know the risk that they pose, should we encounter these fungi, it's the ones that people tend to run the greatest risk.

Magic mushrooms, such as found in the mountains in Australia offer the user the same high as other medicines. In the presence of this kind of mushroom, many sufferers have suffered terrible effects, including death. It's illegal now to possess or use them.

If one doesn't know what they're doing, picking up mushrooms of a field for consumption isn't the best idea. This was evident in Canberra in 1912 when an Chinese cook spotted certain mushrooms that resembled those found in China.

He cooked it as a meal to guests from his circle who were staying. Unknowingly, they were served one of the most deadly mushroom species that is the snowy cap mushroom. They passed away in the hospital for a couple of days.

Amanita phalloides (poisonous mushroom)

Fungi can be found in more than 100,000 species and, as such they are not considered to be plants as per the taxonomy research study. Their spores can be able to survive extreme temperatures, and they can be extremely harmful, in the same way that we know about mould particularly in buildings.

The most efficient way for managing their use is to stay clear of contact with them and instead purchase them from secure suppliers. If you are enticed to choose one in a specific area, the customer should be aware of the things they're doing.

Amanita Pantherina is a type of mushroom.

How to recognize a SHROOM

The psilocybin mushrooms look different from the ordinary dried mushrooms. They are slender, long stalks that are whitish-grey with dark brown caps, with a hint of brown or white at the middle.

Dry mushrooms have a rusty brownish appearance with isolated areas of off-white. Magic mushrooms can be consumed, mixed in meals or used to make tea. They can also be mixed with tobacco or cannabis and then smoked.

Liquid psilocybin is a possibility as it is the natural psychoactive drug that is used in freedom capsules. This liquid appears clear brown and is contained in a tiny vial.

What is the reason people are using the MAGIC MUSHROOMS?

Magic mushrooms are hallucinogenic substances, that when used causes one to experience as well as experience sensations that appear real, but aren't. Magic mushrooms' effects are varied and are believed to be affected by environmental conditions.

The world of mushrooms has a long tradition of being associated with spiritual experience and discovery of self. A lot of people believe that natural drugs like magical mushrooms, bud and mescaline are holy herbs that help people to achieve higher spiritual levels. Others choose magic mushrooms to experience a sense of euphoria or connection or a bizarre perception of time.

The psilocybin found in mushrooms is transformed into psilocin inside the body. It also could affect serotonin levels inside the brain, leading to strange and altered perceptions. The effects can take 20 to 40 minutes to kick in and last up to 6 hours, exactly the same time required for psilocin's metabolism and eliminated.

Many variables influence what magic mushrooms do to you such as age, dose weight, personality, health, the environment and history of mental disease.

Magic mushrooms are often chosen for their psychedelic effects, huge mushrooms have been found to cause anxiety, scary hallucinations, paranoia and confusion at the very least. In actuality most hospital admissions related to the use of magical mushrooms have been related to what's been described as"a "bad excursion." We'll look at its usage in the next section.

The Extent of Use

In from the U.S., the National Survey on Drug Use and Health (NSDUH) revealed that from 2009 to 2015 around 8.5 percent of Americans were psilocybin-positive at a specific time during their day-to-day lives.

People today use psilocybin is a popular activity at dance clubs or with a select group of people seeking an alternative to a religious experience.

Within clinical environments, doctors have examined psilocybin for used to treat cluster headaches, cancer at the end of its stage depression, stress with other disorders of stress.

However, scientists have also questioned the effectiveness of this treatment and its security as a cure.

Chapter 2: Impacts Of Psilocybin Mushrooms

People who had previously been treated using psilocybin had more positive experiences than those who the treatment was a first. The size of the group and dosage, preparation and expectation were key drugs that influence the drug reaction. In general, people in groups that exceeded eight persons found the group to be less welcoming as well as their experience was less enjoyable. However small groups (less than six people) were more welcoming. People also experienced positive drug reactions in these groups. Leary and his colleagues suggested that psilocybin can increases suggestibility, which makes individuals more responsive to social interactions and the environment. In a follow-up review, Jos Ten Berge (1999) which concluded that climate, dose and the context were crucial elements in determining the results of studies that examined the impact of psychedelic drugs on the creativity of artists. A variety of psychological symptoms may be felt during the consumption of psilocybin. These include disorientation, lethargyand giddiness as well as euphori

50

anticipation, depression and euphoria. In one study in which 31% of the participants who were given a high dose of the drug reported feeling of fear of the extreme and 17% experienced intense anxiety. According to Johns Hopkins studies, negative experiences were not common for those who received moderate doses (but nonetheless sufficient to "give the highest chance of experiencing an experiencing a pleasant and extreme experience") while 1/3 of those who received the dose that was high felt anxious or fear.

The low doses of hallucinogens can cause hallucinatory symptoms. Closed-eye hallucinations can be experienced when a person is able to see multicolored geometric shapes as well as creative and imaginative series. People may experience synesthesia, such as sensory experiences when they see different colors. In higher doses, psilocybin may cause "Intensification of affective responses and enhanced ability to reflect as well as relapses of primitive and childlike thinking, as well as stimulation of complex memory trails with significant emotions." The hallucinations that occur in the open eye are not uncommon but they can also be highly specific however they are rarely misinterpreted as reality. A study done in 2011 conducted by Roland R. Griffiths and colleagues indicates that a single large dose of Psilocybin may result in long-term improvements to the customer's personality. About half of study participants -- who were identified as being satisfied, "spiritually committed," and many of them with postgraduate degrees-- demonstrated an improvement in the personality aspect of transparency (assessed by the Revised NEO Personality Inventory) This positive impact was observed for more than a year following the psilocybin experience. According to the study's authors this result is significant since "no study could have demonstrated a change in the personality of healthy adults following an event that was experimentally caused. "[12A second study conducted of Griffiths in 2017 revealed that dosages of 20-30 mg/70 kg of psilocybin, which can cause mystical experiences, caused more lasting positive changes in personality traits, including humility, altruism. While other researchers have also mentioned instances of psychedelic drug usage that has led to new insights into the world of philosophy as well as personal insights however, it's not certain how these findings could be applied to a wider population.

The main phases of a Shroom's journey

The Magic Mushrooms' trip lasts around 3-8 hours. Typically, it takes 4 to 5 hours, based on the dosage and other factors. Other users have noticed subtle variations between the experiences offered by the four primary varieties of 13 psilocibyn based mushrooms and they exhibit similar effects overall, as do the three major levels (installation primary, secondary and the final). The journey begins with physical symptoms (caused via the infusion of adrenaline the body) and are comparable to, but less severe as the consequences of pace, such as dilated pupils larger ears dry mouth, increased breathing, and tension in the muscles. The appetite is typically decreased or eliminated, and vomiting is quite common often leading to vomiting. Even though these physical effects last throughout the journey, when the primary mental effects subside in the middle, they are less noticeable. It is also common for trips to begin in a state of stress release that leads to mumbly conversations (confessing crying, regretting, laughing or crying, etc.). The main stage of the trip usually involves two experiences: periods of disturbed moods and awareness; and visual illusions and pseudo-hallucinations (which you realize are not real)-including intensification of colour moving objects leaving' trails;' entity replications (one cat being many cats); items / scenes being' jumbled up' (rooms with doors on the ceiling); and surreal patterns. Some people may appear very different from the norm and appear amazing, funny or terrifying. You might also hear images or hear noises (known as synaesthesia to understand it). The mood can change from awe to'mongy at ease and anxious, withdrawn and stunned extreme and funny. The mind may become incredibly concentrated on a single subject or overwhelmed by a flurry of thoughts when altering states of consciousness develop. For example: out-of-body sensations (astral projection) as well as time-related fluctuation (slowing or slowing down or stopping) and the divine interaction as well as perceptions (contact with God/nature/'machine Elves'). Ego-related failure can occur in higher levels. It's a sign of our the persona changing or dissolving. in the final part of the experience there is a gradual shift into a normal state of consciousness, typically in " lines', with the illusion that a psychedelic wave rapidly takes over the experience. In this state, participants tend to be quiet and still contemplating the experience. Some suffer from headaches and fatigue.

How many mushrooms will you require to take on your trip?

The chart below shows the dose required for a medium or intense ride. It is not just influenced by the power of mushrooms, or when the mushrooms are dry or dry, but also by previous experiences and tolerance. Regular users be able to develop tolerance (needing more in order to achieve the similar effects) and the effects of mushrooms are fast enough that, after just one week of daily use it is possible that the dose required to feel high would be a risk to the health of. Due to the many variations in the size and amount of water (fresh mushrooms vary between 5 and 90 percent water) It isn't easy to calculate the amount of mushrooms required to walk. The weight of dried mushrooms is a better comparison. However, as the law requires retailers to offer only fresh picked magical mushrooms, it is important to be aware that fresh mushrooms are 10 times as large as dried ones. For every gram that is dried mushrooms is equivalent to 10 grams in fresh shrooms. The strength (or strength) will vary based upon the region from which the mushroom originates and whether they're wild or cultivated (indoor cultivation techniques can greatly enhance the strength).

In this case, the amounts are meant to be dried mushrooms.

What happens to your body after you consume magical mushrooms?

The psilocybin present in shrooms converts into psilocin inside the body. It is believed to alter the levels of serotonin in the brain, which can lead to a variety of abnormal and altered experiences.

The effects can take between 20 and 40 minutes to kick in and last for up to 6 hours, which is about the same length of time that it takes to metabolize psilocin and eliminated. There are many factors that affect how magic mushrooms affect you such as age, dose and the weight and the state of mind, temperament as well as climate and mental health history. After the magic mushrooms are consumed they are digested by both the stomach and the intestinal tract. Additionally, the active ingredients are partially transformed within the liver (e.g. Psilocin transforms into psilocybin) before being transferred onto the heart organs of the lung to allow transport to brain. Psilocin functions similarly in the brain as LSD by increasing a specific kind of serotonin (5HT-2A) that is which is a neuromodulator that regulates certain neurotransmitters, as well as affecting mental processes like mental attitude, vision and memory, as well as consciousness and appetite. However, muscimole is the primary product offered by Fly Agaric affects brain cell receptors for muscarine, which alters levels of acetylcholine GABA and glutamateneurotransmitters in the process of thinking, voice, learning and emotional. This is why Liberty cap and Travel Agaric create different kinds of trips.

What would a magical experience be like?

Your character, experience and temperament, together with the location you will have an impact on the kind of trip you will receive. The dose is equally important and hallucinations that are full-blown can occur with more powerful doses. Every magic mushroom experience is unique according to the way the effects of each drug differ from one. While on the same ride you might be an instant telling a story to a friend and the next, you'll be in an alternate world of your experiences. One thing you should be aware of is that tripping not just a joke. It's as simple as going to the movie and paying for your tickets and then watching a film. One good way to illustrate the concept is the horse tripping and then stepping into a spooky landscape. The horse can guide you to wherever it wishes and take you up and down into valleys, racing for miles, or eating and grazing or even running around in circles. Instead, you can ride the reins and lead the horse through the parts of the landscape you feel most comfortable riding with your own pace and with your own style. The more focused your mind is in addition to the greater amount of time you spend planning for your journey in advance, the more likely you'll be in control of the horse, instead of taking control of yourself. The tripping experiences on the four psilocin-based psilocin-based Fly Agaric are listed below. What they do are all in the same way, and that separates these in comparison to LSD as well as prescription hallucinogens is that the experiences they produce are more likely to bring emotional, loving and moist feelings that are trance-like or dreamy states; supernatural and spiritual experiences; as well as real organic' visions' such animals' faces images of plants, or imaginary creatures.

What are the signs of a bad trip?

Certain negative experiences can be provoked by terrifying dreams (e.g. seeing'monsters'), while others focus on a swell of'repressed angry' (bad feelings squashed at the back of your head because you were unable to manage these feelings). Perhaps the primary reason for negative experiences is the loss of your ego', which is a change in your personal self-image. It can be a traumatic event ("I decided to look around and see what I see") or something that can be a source of anxiety for some. However, bad experiences with magical mushrooms are rare and typically occur in instances of being anxious or agitated or thinking about the implications while going on a trip; or being in a situation that isn't familiar or encountering a negative situation (e.g. accidents) during a trip or making the first trip or getting spiked.' A majority of riders can' get through to the end without much trouble. However, what triggers a horrendous trip to spiral into chaos and cause the full force of a psychotic episode. It's similar to trying to escape away from the Chinese finger puzzle with a simple pull. The more you pull, the bigger it gets. It also affects how you manage bad experiences.

How much will you need to purchase?

Aproximately 1 to 3 grams of dried Mushrooms to get moderate effects on the psyche, up to around 4-7 grams for an entire trip. Averaging less than 1 grams of dried mushrooms will result in an easy excursion. Based on the freshness and drying technique, the amount of fresh psilocybe mushroom can be anywhere from 2 to six times more with between 2 to 20 grams for a moderate journey and up to 8 grams an intense excursion.

Harmful results

There's not a specific reaction to magical mushrooms in relation to the negative effects people experience from drugs like pace, cocaine, and alcohol. People often feel uneasy or confused the next day following a trip, but serious physical or mental indicators are very unlikely. flashbacks -- the memory of returning to the trip days to months later are not uncommon, and tend to be short-lived, one-off and relatively easy to manage whenever they occur. Magic mushroom psychoses are uncommon. They are similar to those of paranoid schizophrenia and are typically seen in those suffering from mental illness-related family history. The difference is that psychoses caused by drugs generally disappear within a couple of weeks provided that the individual isn't taking any drugs. The primary result of consuming mushrooms, particularly flying Agaric memory, is that it quickly disappears after such bizarre experiences.

Pharmacology

Chemistry. Psilocybin (PY, 4-phosphoryloxy-N, N-dimethyltryptamine) is the main psychoactive principle of hallucinogenic mushrooms. Following ingestion, psilocybin gets transformed into the active pharmacological form, the psilocin. Psilocin is also present in the mushrooms, however in less in quantities.

Chapter 3: The Species Of Magic Mushrooms

In varying amounts in more than 200 different species in Basidiomycota and Basidiomycota mushrooms, Psilocybin developed from the ancestor of its species, Muscarine, some 10 to 20 million years ago. In a 2000 study on the global distribution of psilocybin fungi, Gaston Guzan and colleagues looked at the distribution in these genera

* Psilocybe (116 species)

* Gymnopilus (14)

* Panaeolus (13)

* Copelandia (12)

* Pluteus (6)

* Inocybe (6)

* Conocybe (4)

* Panaeolina (4)

* Gerronema (2)

* Agrocybe (1)

* Galerina (1)

Guzman increased his estimate of the number of psilocybin-containing Psilocybe to 144 species in 2005.

Liberty Cap Aka Fairy Mushrooms

About 200 years ago, E. Brande gave the details of London's bizarre incident of poisoning by mushrooms. On the 3rd of October 1799, a poor family harvested and cooked some mushrooms in St. James Green Park. Then, shortly after taking the mushrooms in, the father and four children experienced vomiting symptoms like dilation of pupils, nausea and delusions. The progression of symptoms is thought to be fluid, with in and out decreasing power cycles. In many cases, the image of the father's face was obscured and everything around him appeared dark. This was a frightening vision he believed to signal the imminent death of his son. Two family members (ages between 12-18) consumed small quantities from cooked mushroom, their toxicity outcomes were similar to those seen in family members who had consumed significantly more. The auditory and mental problems were reduced after a couple of hours, and then went away without any adverse effects. Treatments for acute symptoms required emetic therapy and tonic-enhancing. These treatments were hailed as the key cure to "healed" populations. It's very difficult and, in some cases, impossible to gather complete and precise information on all aspects of the history of magic mushrooms from current sources. This is therefore an indication of rare luck and an opportunity to present to historians of mushrooms. Brande's description of normal psilocybin disorder was bolstered with the help of J. Sowerby, creator of "Colour Illustrations of British Mushrooms" (London 1803). Sowerby's book contained a description along with a detailed description of species that caused the case of poisoning that was mentioned in the book by Brande In the spirit of the book by Sowerby the only variety of mushrooms that are distinguished by their cone-shaped caps were believed to cause toxicity . This illustration is typical Psilocybe semilanceata depiction. The genus of this mushroom was referred to by the name of "Agaricusglutinosus Curtis" by his contemporaries of the time and its descriptions are completely compatible with current knowledge regarding Psilocybe semilanceata. A couple of years after, Swedish mycologist E. Fries wrote in "Observationes Mycologicae" (1818), Fries called the genus "Agaricuss in emilanceatus."

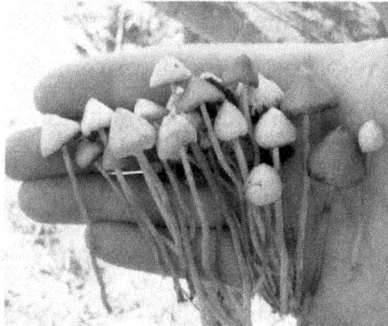

The same fungus has also appeared earlier, as Coprinariuss emilanceatus. and Panaeoluss emilanceatus. Only in 1870 did Kummer and Quelet classified this mushroom as a Psilocybe species. Thus, the literature has two names that are valid: Psilocybe semilanceata (Fr.) Kumm. Or

Psilocybe semilanceata Quel. M. In the year 1900, C. Cooke reported in England three or two recent reports of accidental poisoning with mushrooms. It is interesting that Cooke discovered that only a few mushrooms believed to be blue (var. caerulescens) produced symptoms. The mycologist was the first to ask whether a blue version of this plant is poisonous, or whether environmental triggers caused the bluish color, which caused changes to their chemical structures of the mushrooms which made it poisonous. New discoveries Early discovery A personal kinship to Mexico's psychoactive fungi. Psilocybe semilanceata is a fungus which resembles Psilocybe Semperviva Heim & Cailleux along with Psilocybe Mexicana Heim. Likethem, Mexican species, these thrive in pastures and meadows. A common feature of these species is their calming and slow bluing reactions. The recognition of these similarities to Mexican organisms has sparked interest among scientists seeking to know what else they could know about Psilocybe species that are found in Europe. A team consisting of A. Hofmann, R. Heim started analyzing Psilocybe semilanceata specimens along together with C. Furrer, a mycologist who was studying fruiting organisms throughout Switzerland as well as France. Since 1963, analysis of paper chromatography was able to provide some historical data. Scientists first verified the presence of 0.25 percent psilocybin within dried Psilocybe semilanceata strains. Evidence collection was a remarkable achievement since psilocybin was previously never been discovered in an European species of the genus. Prior to this there was no evidence that only Psilocybe species that are native in Europe, Asia, and North America identified the alkaloid. While Psilocybesemilanceata was not recognized as an important psychoactive species until the 1960s, many daily German-language mycology guide books published before 1963 included species descriptions. Figure 10 provides examples of two accounts that are similar that date from 1962, and the other one from 60 years before. Notice that the 1962 version describes Psilocybesemilanceata as a "worthless" animal-a somewhat incongruous conclusion likely to amuse readers today. On the other hand reports and reports of England cases of poisoning by mushrooms were not incorporated into the mycological literature of Germany. Several authors, Michael & Schulz (1927) and A. Ricken (1915) sent outstanding and practical Psilocybesemilanceata definitions, but these are exceptions very than law. A definition of Psilocybesemilanceata from 1977 shows less focus at specifics and a rather cursory approach to species differentiation, save for specific evidence on microscopic characteristics of the mushroom. In the years 1967 and 1969, an German aquarelle sculpture comprising five fruiting bodies illustrates the habits that the mushroom has in an incredibly realistic manner. In the earlier (1977), Michaelis found alkaloid levels in samples taken in Germany. Since the end of the 1970s researchers in a variety of countries have utilized state-of-the art methods (High-Performance Liquid Chromatography) to examine samples and determine the alkaloid levels. The following articles offer extensive explanations and interpretations of these research studies. Psilocybesemilanceata has become Europe's psychotropic mushroom crop. The diversity is thriving across all over the European continent, prompting intense research efforts.

Psilocybe semilanceata is one of Europe's most commonly used psychoactive fungus. Guzman's monograph from 1983 suggests that Psilocybe semilanceata may be the most widely used psychoactive psilocybe fungus. Although the species is believed to thrive throughout Europe, North America, Australia and Asia Many countries haven't yet studied or identified mycofloras. Therefore, we cannot yet know the prevalence worldwide in Psilocybe semilanceata. However, evidence of this fungus have been reported from the countries listed below located in Europe: Finland, Norway, Sweden, Denmark, Germany, Switzerland, Austria and The Netherlands, Belgium, France, Russia, Poland, Hungary, Romania, Scotland, Wales, Italy and Spain. Unfortunately, there are no maps that accurately describe the pattern of distribution of the animals. In the past, mycologists have ignored tiny animals such as Psilocybe semilanceata that appear to have ecosystems that are shared with others, more widespread species. The skeptical expression "Mushrooms thrive wherever mycologists are" is especially relevant to the Psilocybe Genus. Since the discovery of psilocybin the Genus Psilocybe has been a mystery in the scientific literature, shrouded in the darkness. Stalks usually are by themselves, and typically grouped together, up to 4 inches high and length of goose quill thread color whitish, nearly flat The tube is extremely slim, glutinous; ring at the bottom barely noticeable. "Cap Cap," one up to 2 inches wide and brown in color; fully. Convex, hemispherically developed, and generally glutinous. packed with warmth, it's browner and transparent, sometimes streaked. "Gills multiple single, of the color brownish-purple, which is cloudy; total of twenty horizontal, three smaller ones positioned between them. They discharge the powder in a brownish-purple hue." On its usage it is only said "There is nothing bitter or unpleasant in its flavor however its appearance doesn't suggest it to those who are mushroom enthusiasts." The cap is generally conical to bell-shaped with an obtuse or pointed center with a protrusion that resembles a wart at first; caps tend to be bigger than wide. The margins are bent

, and then curving inwards; later caps are 1.5-4 millimeters wide. Hygrophic, the color is dirty olive-brown when wet, with clear border lines. The color in the center is greenish or ocher against an overall color of pale yellow smudgy and, often, greenish stains. the margins are only bounded along the edges by the dark, watery line. There are no markings or bands visible after drying completely. Without a hood, caps are thin-fleshedand smooth with a pellicle that remains gelatinous and sticky for a lengthy period and then becomes glossy after being cold. Gills range from olive brown to purple-brown with the edges white. The gill's size is quite large The gill connections are generally linear or and up to 3.5 millimeters wide, attached to stems only, and then completely disengaged. Spores are smooth and with an elliptical shape, measuring 12-16 u by 6-8,u. Spore dust is blackish-purple-brown. The stem is tiny that is almost evenly small and bent, 6-12cm long and 12.5-2 mm thick and yellowish or whitish. the areas that are stressed develop blueish-green staining. Stems are silky smooth , and slightly loose in the middle. cortinate fibrils show up in the form of traces of a shawl that is porous and stuffed with a white wool-like fibrous thread. The flesh of the cap is pale yellow in dry form and the stem's flesh turns ocher brown, especially downwards. It's smellless and moderately sour. The fungus is active in the months of August through October usually in gregarious groups, and can be found in fields and along pathways which feed on dung that is completely broken down. It's not uncommon.

Mycologists concentrate on researching Psilocybes but Psilocybe semilanceata is a well-known and widely known Psilocybes species. In addition, those who are interested in mushrooms who's interest are not strictly scientific will typically not maintain their publications in the form charting distribution. There is however one diagram from 1986 showing the pattern of distribution of Psilocybe semilanceata across Germany. There is hardly any written information about the locations that Psilocybe kinds are found in the eastern region of Germany. On my excursion, I observed Psilocybe semilanceata in various areas, like close to my home town of

Mansfeld in The Vorharz Mountains, in the Duben marshlands and other eastern German marshlands. Friends that are mycologists also have told me about mushrooms found throughout the countryside. A 1952 book is one of the few books that contain descriptions of mushrooms found in the southeastern part of Saxony. Psilocybe populations thrive faster on moist pastures, that are surrounded by woods. Based on my experience, Psilocybe semilanceata grows in the majority of German woodlands. The it produces fruit between late September and October. This favors acidic soils and grassy slopes within or around woodlands. The plants are usually grouped in groupings that contain 30 or less mushrooms. Deer droppings and other animal manure can be located there, but mushrooms seldom grow right on top of dung. Sometimes, extremely stunted specimens are found along the roadsides on the mountains. In the cow pastures of older times soil provides a perfect environment for mycelial growth that is extensive. Certain areas have wide areas yield abundant fruiting bodies, which mirror the amount of mycelial growth within the soil. If there is enough moisture, optimal yields are possible provided the field is fed at least one time during the weeks prior to the season of fruiting. However, mushrooms also thrive on sheep and horse pastures in normal conditions. These grassy areas in forests are usually the nursery grounds of deer providing additional nutrients for the vegetation. Psilocybe semilanceata however, doesn't grow in areas in areas where artificial fertilizers were employed. These pastures are also bordered by water-saturated creeks or swamplands. In summer, the temperatures that are warm in these areas creates a perfect setting for the development of mycelial mycelial. In Germany the environment of the mushroom is varied from mountainous to coastal areas in which the species was discovered at altitudes of up to 1,720 meters (5,160 feet) over sea levels (MTB-8443 1985). A sample was collected from the former Czechoslovakia at altitudes that ranged between 330 and 1,000 meters (1,000-3,000 feet) in one spot at 1,400 meters (4,200 feet) over sea level. Based on the distribution patterns the species don't appear to be averse to a specific altitude. As of the year 1986 there were

44 sites recorded in the former Czechoslovakia which yielded 54 specimens. Unlike other mushroom species, such as cultivated commercial white mushrooms (Agaricusbisporis), Psilocybesemilanceata can bear fruit in a comparatively broader temperature range. Although Psilocybesemilanceata is widespread across Germany, this does not seem to favor specific areas where it occurs in marked abundance or density. One major obstacle to the development of the species is the limited availability of fertilizers in areas that are suitable for the mushroom to flourish. It's likely that's the reason the species hasn't adapted into different ecosystems within Germany in the last few decades. The descriptions of the level in earlier papers are similar to the current observations.

At times, Psilocybe semilanceata may develop huge numbers of fruiting bodies at certain locations where the conditions for growth are favorable. All Lake and Dam Marshlands .... Fantastic 8'/2! In the present I'd like to add more information concerning two marshland locations which we have studied for mycological ground analyses over the last few years. In a slightly acidic area the fruiting bodies formed within a grassy valley within a very high grass. This was in a zone that was surrounded by a lake as well as an aquisitor pool. In areas that are exposed to intense sunlight, temperatures are much higher than neighboring regions, which was the case all through the fall. Deer droppings are a common source of fertilization. The fruiting bodies of the first harvest at this site that contained mushrooms were covered with stems that were up to 81/2 inches. [! (21,5 cm) tall, extremely tall grass that was very thick that was growing in the field. Mushroom caps were so small that easy identification of species as Psilocybesemilanceata was not immediately feasible. Following a bluing reaction the chromatography study was needed to verify the organisms. But, the subsequent discoveries led to species that could be identified localally based on their morphological traits. We collected 30-60 specimens every fall for three years. Unfortunately, the site was destroyed by man-made alteration to the marshlands, as well as the building of an entry road. The same time, we walked to an additional area about one mile away in distance from our first. The field was extremely wide and was and was an ancient cow-pasture, which was frequently was grazed. It was located along a river which completely soaked the earth. Sheep are still grazing in the fields and deer dung is generally discovered in the hay. Psilocybe semilanceata can be found in abundance. Each autumn thousands of fruitsing body fill the field. We visited this field 3 times each autumn for three years, and collected over 2,800 mushrooms (about 140 grams or 5 pounds dry weight) on the farm. While some fruiting bodies could be seen clearly on the grassy soil but the vast majority of the organisms were enclosed in grass clumps. When it is dry, Psilocybe semilanceata is a well-known plant. The fruiting bodies are very hypertrophic, and that is why the caps' color change to a dark dark olive when the mushroom is hot. It was only by careful observation of the gills and bent stems helped us discern between the wet ones as well as the Panaeolus species. Unlike other species of psychotropic mushrooms one of the main characteristics that distinguishes Psilocybe semilanceata's coloration is blue. on the cap and lower part on the stem. The bodies that produce fruit are old and wet. may produce random blue, clear stains on their caps. On the other hand, stem discoloration doesn't occur until the bodies that produce fruit are separated from the mycelia for 30-60 minutes. Even in areas of high production, along with other areas there are mushrooms with blueish-green discoloration that did not exhibit this characteristic. Through the drying process the blue coloring remains however some fades may occur. Psilocybe semilanceata's descriptions of its history are extremely detailed, and I'm unable to provide any information of superior quality. In spite of various views in the literature in opposition there is a distinct scent emanating from exposed damp fruiting bodies. The odor is similar but not as strong as the one associated with Psilocybe bohemica. It is usually described as a resemblance to radishes and poppies, however it is not usually unpleasant.

In addition, they have a distinctive characteristic that is not found in any other species. Psilocybe semilanceata mushrooms change into quartz-illuminated. The individual responsible for this incident is not at the time of this writing.

Psilocybe semilanceata is perhaps the most potent psychoactive mushroom in those of the European species. The amazing sophistication and speedy appearance of symptoms were evident in my various psychotic experiences. The same components form in the account that describes the first self-experiment by mycologist. After ingestion of 1.3 grams (less than one sixth of an ounce) in dried crushed mushrooms (30 mushrooms in total) in water with an unfulfilled stomach 20 minutes passed until the sudden appearance of hallucinatory symptoms, such as intense tears. The visions are more accurately described as a combination of visual thoughts. Later, in the writings I was introduced to the term "visualization." I experienced a terribly disturbing daydream-like trip, during which I was snatched by a witch... We three went to different places at times. Prior to that, everything that I was living with seemed dull and washed. It was like I "read" abstract patterns while closed my eyes with no noticeable light as well as emotional impact. A floating dysphoria arose, accompanied by thoughts of guilt. The symptoms ceased abruptly within five hours and were then and then a gradual onset of mild headaches, but no other side effects were noted.

On the other hand an experiment with about half of the earlier dose stood out due to an influx of memories and a experience of emotions from youth, and also some strange sensations of merging and melting In the late summer, I was taking walking in the woods and I took 0.6 grams of pulverized mushrooms. The weather was pleasant and sunny and I strolled through wide open spaces close to my home in which I played when I was a kid. At first, I was struck by an emotional experience that can be described by a child's fascination and wonder at the forest nearby. The surroundings seemed to be to be in stark contrast and my impressions of the environment seemed fresh and unadulterated. After a while, I remembered in great detail how tiny the trees had been decades earlier and that, even before midnight, I'd never witnessed any other development in the plant life that I was afraid of. My body movements sound more natural and child-like. This incredible reliving of my childhood lasted for about two hours. When I returned home I saw a small calves in the field. The calf caused a amount of anxiety within me when I realized the sly nature of it. The love for the animal led to a short mixed encounter and the cow. I found it to be very bizarre and uncomfortable. The effects subsided after 4 hours, with no further adverse effects.

A third experiment using Psilocybe semilanceata found in Oregon brought about a complete name-calling experience with a 19th century person and we gathered a substantial quantity of "liberty caps" in a field close to Astoria. Then, when we returned to our hotel, I consumed the freshest of six mushrooms. The main reason for my subsequent encounter was a 19th-century elegant lady's watercolor drawing which caught my attention completely. Then I realized I was living in a previous life which began with my birth within Germany around 1813. I was Alexander Schmitt, I thought I had died in 1871. I emigrated into North America with my parents and other immigrants when I was young boys. While in America, in U.S., 1 changed my name to Smith.

I lived in a small Kentucky town that was called Sharpville also known as Shopville. My life was filled with contradictions , and I drank plenty of alcohol. My needs mirror my own life that included beating my wife and treating her like the tyrant I was. The more the incident grew I completely identified with Alexander Smith. In those days I was completely unaware of my native German and my thought processes were in English. In the end, I was experiencing the final moments of Alexander Smith's life. I was lying on a lot of white sheets in a hospital exhausted. When I woke up, I realized my wife murdered me in order to bring an end to her adolescent assaults over the many years. I was convinced that I wouldn't live for long. I'm likely to die. Fortunately, the battle was over before I had to face the ultimate battle with death. Three years later the unforgettable event is still burning into my brain. The impact on my mind from the event hasn't diminished. Similar findings to earlier manifestations could cannot be explained using Contemporary scientific principles. In any case, a systematic effort to determine the truthfulness and authenticity of the places and people that were involved. The person who was witness to the above events had never visited Kentucky or even knew whether or not the town of Sharpville or Shopville was actually a reality and never had any interest about the U.S. region. In spite of his purely atheistic background, he was never able to find the same experiences as possible. S. However Grof detailed a series of unique events and stated that they could happen very frequently when under the influence of hallucinogens. He also observed that these instances aren't common as many people have hallucinogenic drug applications.

In closing this section I'd be pleased to offer a brief account of an experience which demonstrates how the effects of psychotropic substances can vary between individuals, depending on the context where the experience is experienced. After taking 0.6 milligrams of pulverized mushrooms inside orange juice within about thirty minutes the effects started to show in an endless sequence of pictures that could not be seen with closed eyes. However, there were no clear emotions of euphoria or dysphoria were observed; the reaction to these photos can be better described as "temporary delight". The initial images of entangled ornaments changed as time passed and transformed into plants that had strange, unrealized features that were not present on Earth. I believed that these photos reflect my long-standing fascination with plants. But, when I saw a mirror in front of me, I saw "a dark-looking man with a squinty eye." Then I realized, slowly, that this thought was my own mental state and that I rarely found it easy to "see what's behind the façade."

The analysis instructions was a confirmation of my findings. This was a new issue before. Countries, along with Switzerland and the former Czechoslovakia were the main focus of research. It was discovered that the study of different dried mushrooms to study alkaloid production gave an average of 1 percent dry weight psilocybin regardless of the country of origin. The subject of chemical racism was arousingly addressed in other species like the fly agaric mushrooms. While, unlike plants in the higher types of mushrooms this pattern hasn't been proven yet.

The evidence does not support the idea of a species ' chemical composition can differ significantly between samples. Psilocybe semilanceata as well as Inocybe Aeruginascens are the two species that have the least amount of variation in psilocybin levels across different samples.

Psilocybe Cyanescens - Powerful Mushrooms Growing On Wood Debris

There is at least one Psilocybe population is present in Europe with the exception of Psilocybe semilanceata. In this context I'll point out that there is a lot of disagreement between eminent taxonomists on the distinction of one species within the Genus Psilocybe. For instance, various methods for separating the Genus Hypholoma in the same way as the Genus Stropharia exist. In the event that Psilocybe semilanceata has a name which has been for a long time clearly defined and is easily known by this name There are, according to Krieglsteiner other blue-colored mushrooms that could be classified as part of the "Psilocybe complex cyanescens."

They all thrive on soils that are not treated as well as plants waste. Based on current information these terms are simply synonyms for Psilocybe Cyescens Wakefield emend. Krieglsteiner: herbariums. The problem is that Psilocybe macroscopically-described descriptions are not well defined and frequently overlap. Therefore, further mycological research on Psilocybe cyanescens are needed. To accomplish this new mushroom extracts from different European regions should be utilized as well as biochemical methods in the investigation. However, Guzman's division of Psilocybe Cyanescens cyanescens according to geographic region was not accurate. According to his Method-Psilocybemairei was home to North Africa when Psilocybe cyanescens was found in England, and Psilocybeserbica allegedly grew in Serbia and Bohemia. The distribution of the whole species appears to cover an extensive area, with differences in temperature and geographic sites. The morphologies of these species are diverse and should be anticipated when dealing in a relationship with "fresh" species or species that are not yet established themselves but continue to expand across new regions. The map below shows the places within Europe in Europe and North Africa where different herbarium extracts of Psilocybe Cyanescens were discovered. But, Psilocybe microscopic details are not well defined and can often overlap. Thus, additional mycological studies for Psilocybe cyanescens are required. In this regard fresh samples of mushrooms from a variety of European regions should be utilized and biochemical methods are also included to investigate.

A description of any fungus specific species can be valid when the sample's Latin diagnosis is reported in a journal of mycology as well as the distinctive characteristics of the other mushrooms. The year 1946 was when Wakefield identified Psilocybe cyanescens Wakefield a group of blue dark-spored fungi that was discovered in Kew in England's botanical gardens. The fungi were intended to develop spontaneously, i.e. the spores were imported from overseas along together with other plant material. These mushrooms are found frequently in botanical gardens and the imports are likely to occur if the specific mushroom was not previously observed within the vicinity. Gymnopiluspurpuratus could be added to other areas (see the section 3.5). Mushrooms showed a much stronger blue staining response than Psilocybesemilanceata. They were seen growing over a period of time on tiny pieces of wood within Kew Gardens forest areas during the fall time. One of the most striking characteristics of these mushrooms are their undulating and curved eyes. Guzman states that the species found within British Columbia and the United States ' Pacific Northwest (Northern California, Oregon, Washington) are similar to the ones located within Kew Gardens (see Figure 24). The macroscopic information and photos are identical to the mushroom species found in England. Only DNA analyses and cross-breeding studies using single-spore mycelia will provide definitive evidence of identification. I'll continue to build on this stage in the future. The year 1975 was the first time Holland was able to find fruiting organisms of this species. In 1972, additional blue mushrooms that were growing in a crowded manner on lawn and decaying of reeds were discovered throughout the Swiss Jura Mountain (MTB 8511). Some samples were collected in Austria's Steiermark field during the fall of the year 1976, and also in Corsica's Mediterranean island in the years 1972 and 1984. Numerous fruiting bodies that were identified to be Psilocybe cyanescens have also been found at various times in Germany More details about the various specimens can be found below On October 31, 1983, large amount in fruiting organisms were discovered within the lower parts within Bavaria (MTB 7542). They were surrounded by grass. The mushrooms were discovered over a 100-yard area close the old dump, forming colonies. Some were tiny, larger ones and partially interspersed. They were found scattered through decaying plant materials, including seeds, twigs and even mulch. They were green, and clearly blue, with an icy blue hue near the edge of the base. Some fruiting bodies produced blue stains upon the treatment even when it was at low temperatures. What is the definition for Psilocybe cyanescens in the following paragraphs is slightly simplified, however it is a common reference to other collections. The sizes and dimensions may differ the caps are 5-40 millimeters wide, conic in the beginning and with co-ordinate fibrils rising up to the stem before fading quickly, becoming bell-shaped earlier and an umbo that is sharp. Later, they expand to plane with waves or undulating edges tiny remnants of caps, typically convex in older species of mushrooms.

Deep brown chestnut when it is fresh and damp, it fades to blue-green to blue-blue color after it has dried. Gills: Attachment is close subdecurrent, color to dirty beige in the early stages and then changing to a the color of cinnamon-purple due to the spore maturation. Blue staining reaction due to the pressure can be normal. Stem: 30-85mm long, 1.5-3 mm thick. Mycelial fibers and stems change color if blue stains do not exist. Odor: similar to onions or rice. Spars: 6-8x 9-14 u. Within the year 1976, blueing mushrooms found on plant debris was found in the German Saarland district. A number of sets are directly from Southern Black Forest (MTB 7515 1959, 1963,) as well as the Vogtland (1979) as well as Rheinland (MTB 4706 1982). Similar mushrooms were discovered close to Hamburg (MTB 2428 1983) and Bremen (1982 1983). These are especially intriguing because the greenhouses in these communities of Rhododendron Park as well as the People's Park in those communities have been dotted with wood chips during the fall which enabled the mushrooms to grow more frequently (thousands of mushrooms) than what we normally see in the areas around and where the organisms are thriving in various locations. The findings of these communities more than likely confirm the existence of an introduced species similar to this since it requires access to mycelia to the colder autumn temperatures. Many wood-chipdwelling species have been reported from the Pacific Northwest of the U.S., such as Psilocybestundi, Psilocybebaeocystis, Psilocybepelliculosa, and others (see also Section 7.1). PsilocybeMurr'scaerulescens. The species is also from Mexico. Wasson's very first Psilocybe mushroom to be recorded as psychoactive during his own experiment on June 29th 1955. It is not known much about the collection's chemical composition. I studied a few of the mushrooms from the collections of Rheinland Germany back in the year 1989. The reports were as follows the following: psilocybin 0.51 percent in dried mushroom Psilocin: 0.08% of dried mushrooms Baeocystin 0.04 percent of dried mushrooms Other analyses of German mushrooms produced similar results. These amounts were within the Mexican species ' range of alkaloid concentrations. In the past Czechoslovakia in which the mushrooms are commonly referred to as Psilocybebohemica the largest studies of propagation psychoactivity and chemical compounds that comprise the Psilocybecyanescens complex were carried out. Mycelia makes use of various kinds of plant debris , and develops on wet cardboard in which they transform into rhizomorphs, just like they would in nature. Rhizomorphs are mycelial fibers that are thick that contain water and nutrients. Also, we produce serious blueishes.

Hawaiian Myths About this Confusing Mushroom

Reports of accidental infections of dark-spread dung-infesting the mushrooms (Panaeolus genus) across the globe have been reported from at least the beginning of the 19th century. In 1816 in

Hyde Park in London's Hyde Park, a poor man picked what that he believed to be edible, white the mushrooms ("champignons," Agaricusbisporus).

After ingestion of these fungi, the field of vision became blurred. He could only see confusion that was lightheaded and dizzy. The chair fell to the ground. He could feel all his energy lost from his body as he became completely numb to surroundings and never really noticing the place the he was. The effects of dizziness abated while his heart beat decreased until he slept..The effects were then traced the genus "Agaricus campanulatus Linnaeus," confused for champignons by the person who was suffering. A similar genus was also blamed for an identical case of poisoning a year ago. Both accounts cite St. James Green's overdose in 1799 with Psilocybe semilanceata. It's quite plausible, because there are psilocybin producing mushrooms even within the Panaeolus group. The issue is which of the fifteen European organisms produces the psychoactive ingredient remains an issue of major scientific debate. While I am unable to provide an absolute or definitive evidence to answer this question There are a few conclusive conclusions from recent biochemical analyses of mushrooms that have been found in herbariums in which certain species are believed to be deposited. In particular, the other American species belonging to the Panaeolus genus don't appear to be the same as comparable European species.

I'd like to discuss some of the historical instances that demonstrate Panaeolus Intoxication here. A hallucinogenic phenomenon that was traditionally is attributed to Panaeolus papilionaceous. (Bull. : Fr.) Quel's accidental consumption. All over Maine, USA, in 1914. Below is an abbreviated copy of. W.'s statement of impact. On the 10th of July in 1914, one found a beautiful mess of mushrooms (Panaeolus papilionaceous) which was cooked to serve for dinner...Mrs. I've eaten every single one of them. And I'm fine. Strange signs in a brief time.Initially objects change into bizarre bright hues. A field of redtop grass appeared to be a vibrant green and red horizontal stripes. Then a dark gray cloud was spotted across all the land... Then we both began to become amusing, and had an uncontrollable urge to laugh and laugh loudly and sometimes even hysterically... I had a terrible experience. Numerous human faces of all types and shapes however, all of them grotesque appeared to cover the entire room and spread out at a rapid pace, and a lot of them were snatching me off from all sides. They all screamed quickly and horribly, undergoing convulsions, and getting more gruesome. Some of them were upside-down. The faces appeared in a myriad of vibrant and vivid colors. They were so vivid that one could only compare them to flames in the red, purple, green and yellow, as firework displays... The whole event lasted around six hours. The procedure was not a cause of harm. No stomach discomfort or discomfort was observed.

In 1915's winter in 1915, a Panaeolus species appeared accidentally in the New York's greenhouse for mushrooms. The fruiting bodies were mistakenly overwhelmed by the champignons that had been that were produced. This error led to poisoning cases so rare the fact that Murrill identified the fungus as Panaeolus venenosus. It took a while before he learned that the species was earlier classified in the form of Agaricus subbalteatus. & Br. & Br. and Br. Paris 1861. The current mix-phrase, Panaeolus subbalteatus (B.&Br.) Sacc. The first publication was in 1887. Some cases of poisoning with similar symptoms, triggered by Panaeolus species have been reported within both the United States (1917) and Australia (after 1940) and in Australia (after 1940), where the species was identified as "Panaeolus Ovatus Cooke & Massee."

In 1939, in conjunction with Linder's classification experiments, these sources prompted Schultes to write Panaeolussphinctrinus (Fr.) Quel. Teonanacatl mushroom is mentioned in the 17th and 16th centuries of Mexican literature. But, Wasson, Heim and their associates and Singer are unable to identify the Panaeolus mushroom within Mexico as well as their psychoactive Psilocybe report on species. The year 1959 was the first time Guzman declared this species "the false Teonanacatl." To date, in Mexico Guzman has not been able to prove the native use of any Panaeolus species. The indigenous people of

Mexico considered blueing and hallucinogenic Panaeolus mushroom poisonous. Despite England's report of a poisoning incident the early German sources do not classify Panaeolus as poisonous. Similar to how Psilocybe species were seen as. Figure 27 shows the characteristic of the species as well as its habitat. Interpretations of the present are generally more ambiguous and less accurate than the 1927 Michael and Schulz's. In Germany the situation of Panaeolus mushrooms was first documented in the year 1957. Based on the current research it seems that the fungus responsible was likely to be Panaeolus Reticulis (Fr.) Gill. Between 30 and 60 minutes before the consumption of the cooked mushrooms the vision field of the woman began to narrow. In the meantime, her eyes were extremely dilapidated. As soon as she noticed that she was having problems and had an anxiety attack. The entire area was covered by curtains. There were no indicators after the effects subsided. A second Panaeolus subbalteatus toxicosis epidemic took place in Leipzig in the year 1970. Similar to the New York 1915 incident, the mushrooms accidentally arose from a population of commercially produced mushrooms (in this case, Strophariarugoso-annulata Farlow) and were then inadvertently eaten. The definition of the results is unusual. The fungus is found growing in Dung, Waste, and soil Tales of contamination and even the word "dung-inhabiting" mushroom provide clues as to the kind of environments this fungus prefers to flourish in. Sometimes, they grow directly on dung, or on heavily fertilized pastures. Sometimes they are found on garbage heaps compost or straw substrates on which mushrooms are grown commercially. European Panaeolus species that possess Psilocybin possess a distinct characteristic that makes them different from Psilocybe species: they don't produce blue stains after being injured or handled. In his 1977 account of an Scottish incident of intoxication, Watling talks about colored blue hues as well as Panaeolus Subbalteatus's stem caps which formed due to pressure. Blue stains are quite rare as my observations suggest. Additionally, Pacific Northwest U.S. reports have reported that only one in 100 mushrooms turn blue. A topic that is a source of contention in the studies is the species toxic to humans Panaeolus foenisecii (Pers. : Fr.) Kuhn. Formerly was known as Psilocybe and Psathyrella, this fungus is now known as Panaeolina instead of Panaeolus because it's a species that does not thrive on dung, produces fruits only after the harvest of hay and spores which are brownish-purple and rough. But, many Panaeolus species bear black print spores when they are placed on white paper within glass vessels to prevent drying out. However, not all panaeolus foenscecii's seeds (Pers.-Fr.) Kuhn.do grow at the same time, which could cause the gills' appearance to be soiled. Because of taxonomic differentiation problems, there are only a very little information about the exact.

Taxonomic Debate On the 25th of May, 1986 I will present 147 Panaeolus Subbalteatus fruiting bodies in all stages and stages of growth in Heringsdorf located on the East German Sea Coast. They were cultivated on a pile of compost comprised of manure from horses. Contrary to Psilocybe species that are found in springtime, Panaeolus mushrooms are available all through the autumn season. The distinction between

Panaeolus animals is further compromised because they're very hygrophic with caps that can differ from white under whitish or reddish-brown, to extremely dark black-brown. The older mushrooms in the compost heap had cracked-maturity caps, with edges bent upwards and covered with spores. Only two of the mushrooms had blue-colored tops and the stems didn't change color from light to dark. Panaeolus subbalteatus is known as "Panaeolus Variabilis" by the authors of American literature since certain stems mimic the appearance of other species of mushrooms which can cause taxonomic debate. It is also known to be found close to panaeolus foenisecii (Pers. : Fr.) Kiihn. This can open up more opportunities to make mistakes, especially in the event that mushrooms aren't carefully scrutinized. As the Panaeolus subbalteatus mushrooms age, their caps smoothen, which is an important taxonomically-related characteristic. A long and watery margin of the cap is known as the mushroom. Only the psilocybin producing plant will be discussed further below. Recent analyses have revealed that Panaeolus subbalteatus is among the most potent psychoactive European organisms within the Panaeolus group. Ola'h's monograph on the world Panaeolus genus was written in the early 1960s, causing some confusion when he identified certain species as "latent sources of psilocybin." For example, Panaeolusfoenisecii sometimes produces psilocybin. Both Panaeolus species share one characteristic that sets them apart from other species that are discussed throughout the book. They create five-replaced indole compounds like serotonin, and its biochemical counterpart 5hydroxytryptophan. Serotonin is a common chemical found in both mammals and humans. It acts as neurotransmitters in the brain, but it is not clear if the consequences of serotonin are fully realized. But, it must be kept in mind it is true that serotonin and 5-hydroxytryptophan have no effect for oral consumption. If you are conducting thin-layer analysis, psilocin is able to confuse both substances. Incredibly, the reports of Ola'h do not agree with current research as his research has also demonstrated Psilocin's presence within Panaeolus species! The most recent research on specifically chosen European Panaeolus species mushroom material did not reveal significant levels of psilocin found in these samples. "Chem classes" related to species were not identified. I would guess that most accidental intoxications could be caused by the consumption of the subbalteatus Panaeolus, with the exception of one species that has been introduced to the tropical world. It isn't much is known about Panaeolus Reticulis and its distribution zone and its chemical composition.

But, Bremen's overdose shows that the psychoactive nature of this group (see figure 28). Two fruiting bodies were discovered in a field in the year 1985 which had dry weights of 0.03-0.05 percent serotonin and psilocybin. All the characteristics of the mushroom including flesh-colored, wrinkled tops, were in line with Panaeolusretirugis descriptions. Based on his analyzes, Stijve hypothesized that Panaeolussubbalteatus ' dried fruiting bodies contain about 0.1 percent psilocybin, regardless of location, and a small amount of baeocystin. Nonetheless, records of intoxications with predictably high psychoactive effects appear to provide evidence against such small amounts of alkaloids in Panaeolussubbalteatus. In fact dried mushrooms that are found within those in the U.S. Pacific Northwest area have been found to produce 0.16%-0.65 percent of psilocybin. Additionally, the initial research on species of the species in North America (1959) led to the discovery of a water-soluble indole substance which is believed as baeocystin. My research on mycelia and 19 fruiting bodies found at the Heringsdorf site showed psilocybin rates which are completely compatible to U.S. evidence A significant number of synonyms currently used for the species provided by Gerhardt also suggest significant taxonomic uncertainties as well as insufficient coordination and communication of information.

Inocybe Aeruginascens: Fast-Spreading New Arrivals

June 15, 1965, 1. Ferencz discovered fruiting body that were named "fibrehead mushroom" located in Osca, Hungary, Pest County. The characteristics of these mushrooms didn't match the characteristics of any of the known Inocybe family of organisms that were identified in the scientific literature. The same year, and several times in the following years, Ferencz and other mycologists discovered a large number of mushrooms growing in various areas. In 1968 the mushrooms were classified as a new species dubbed Inocybe Aeruginascens Babos.

Strange distribution trends within Hungary in Hungary and Germany In 1985, at 17 sites (46 samples) within Hungary, some mycologists who were specialized in studying the genus Inocybe found greenish-colored fiberheads. In her 1983 paper Babos observed that Inocybe Aeruginascens was now the most common mushroom found in the sandy regions in Budapest's Hungarian capital. The species is known to grow in these environments whether in groups of gregarious individuals on the sandy soils of the poplar forests or in mixed woods that contain poplars. They are often found in meadows surrounding poplar trees. The mushrooms are loyal to the area, and grow each year, creating weather conditions. As of 1975 Kaspar occasionally found the in Berlin's Inocybe species. More detailed studies revealed that mushrooms are often mistakenly identified. In the year 1965 the fruiting bodies of the species were identified. Berlin arboretum (Baumschulenweg). Certain mycologists with no expertise in mushrooms have mentioned that variety "in in passing." There are several varieties (about 160) from the broad European Inocybe genus are unable to be distinguished from each others, and thus receive very only a little attention from mycologists who specialize in. They are part of the large category of mushrooms referred to as "No brown Mushrooms" from American literature, and because of this, they can create major taxonomic issues. Some other types of mushroom that fall into this category include the Panaeolus species as well as Psilocybe genus. When an "new mushroom" is discovered the root of it must be explored. Herink is one of the Czech mycologist, claims to have first discovered this species around 1930. He is the only person to have deposited spores into an herbalist's collection, but the mushroom was never discovered as biochemically-based Inocybe Aeruginascens. Because Inocybe Aeruginascens's fruiting bodies were observed at the same time in Hungary and Germany however, the exact path of migration across the globe of the species was not able to be identified. The species could have initially was restricted to a tiny region and only began to be noticed after moving into new environments. We are unable to predict the possibility of mutations emerging from species we know in a short time. In the 1980s, several fruiting organisms were discovered within Holland (1980) in the Swiss Rhone Valley (Wallis Canton) (1984). The species was a favorite among biochemists and medical professionals right after the release of G from 1983. Drewitz identified a mysterious psychotropic poisoning that these mushrooms caused within Potsdam, Germany, between June and July of 1980. The range of results was extraordinary for Inocybe genus of mushrooms since a variety of species cause the traditional symptoms of muscarine poisoning. Muscarine can cause symptoms like swelling of the pupil (miosis) and a decrease in salivation and production of saliva. Muscarine was found in more than forty Inocybe species. The first records of death after ingestion of active muscarine-containing

InocybepatouillardiBres. In the early 20th century.

Gymnopilus Purpuratus Magnificient Mushrooms from South America

Another literature-documented controversy revolves around the psychoactivity of several Gymnopilus group members. Over 50 years ago an unusual case of toxicity was observed in October 1942and was being attributed to Pholiota spectrumabilis. Today, they were regarded to be Gymnopilus the spectabilis (Fr.) A.H. Smith, USA. Also known as Gymnopilus Junonius (Fr.) Orton across Europe.

A lady was walking in the woods . She she brought a couple of nibbles from an invasive mushroom with the confidence that she would be able to discern edible from poisonous ones. She was able to see the most stunning scenes of color and sounds while lying down however, she did not feel any discomfort. If a woman is experiencing discomfort, is in need of a doctor immediately. In response to questions about my symptoms, I informed her that some of the mushrooms can cause symptoms. I explained that the mushrooms I mentioned were not classified as poisonous nor did they live for long. In the same night, the woman called, and reported that her visions had vanished and she felt normal once more. She said that in the event that this was the best method to die from mushroom poisoning, she would be totally for them.

Another instance of poisoning was documented by Harvard, Massachusetts: at around nine a.m. in the morning of September 9th 1996. A retired mechanical engineer aged 56 picked an assortment of mushrooms gathered on the side of the road, right in the vicinity of his home. The mistaken belief was that they them being honey-colored mushrooms (Armillaria mellea , an edible species) The man tried the fresh flesh and was a bit oily. He then took the mushrooms home, which his wife cleaned and then fried the mushrooms in butter. He consumed up to three or two caps around noon and was exhausted in the afternoon and "woozy" after 15 minutes. His head felt blurred, and his vision became blurred. The room seemed smaller, and the walls appeared less than usual. Things shimmered, then turned bright, with dark areas at the center. The plants and trees were vibrant green, with violet lines. The feelings weren't bad. The lighting seemed artificially dim as if it was a color television picture. Even though he could not gather the thoughts of his mind, his brain was sharp and clear. He asked himself questions and was able to answer them immediately. However, he was unable to find it after putting down the book down.

Within a couple of hours the three participants were able to give a concise account of their experiences. The mushrooms that were involved were described in the category of Pholiota spectabilis. But, this classification is disputed, since it is usually described as having a very bitter taste. There are more species of the Gymnopilus genus Gymnopilus throughout North America (73) than in Europe (15). Mushrooms that are 24 "tall! Although Gymnopilus junionius is among the most massive species of mushrooms (with stems that are observed to grow as high as 24 inches 60 cm] in height) however, there aren't identified

European instances of Gymnopilus species being intoxicated. All Gymnopilus species ' bitter flavor can be a powerful preventative against eating them as table mushrooms However. But, U.S. toxicity events led Hatfield and his coworkers to test the phytochemical properties of some of the animals. Between 1968 and 1971, this research group discovered that eight animals that included Gymnopilus Junonius, had inactive styrylpyrones such as bis-noryangonin. In a different incident that was accidental an incident, a different dispute that has been reported in the literature concerns the psychoactivity of a number of Gymnopilus Genus organisms.

In the past 50 years an uncommon incident of overdose occurred in the month of October 1942, because of Pholiota spectabilis. In the present, they are identified as Gymnopilus spectrumabilis (Fr.)A.H. Smith, USA. Often named Gymnopilus junonius (Fr.) Orton within Europe. In the afternoon, a woman took a stroll in the woods . She ate bites of a mushroom she found, certain that she could distinguish the edible ones from those that were poisonous. The woman began to witness stunning sights of music and colors while lying down but she didn't feel any discomfort. Anyone who thinks she is that she is a specialist must be contacted immediately. When she inquired about her symptoms, i informed her that certain mushrooms have been known to trigger the symptoms. I further explained that the mushrooms I mentioned weren't labeled as poisonous, and they did not last long. The next day, she reached out me and reported that her visions had disappeared and she was completely calm again. She told me that If this was the only method to die from mushroom toxicity, she'd be for it. Another instance of poisoning was reported at Harvard, Massachusetts: on September 9, 1966 about 9 a.m.

The former mechanical engineer from Harvard, who was 56 years old, Massachusetts, gathered a collection of mushrooms that were arranged along the road in the front of his home. Based on the false notion of them being honey-colored mushrooms (Armillaria Mellea is an edible species) The man savored the fresh flesh and found that it was bitter, but the mushrooms were brought home and his wife cleaned them and cooked them in butter. He ate between two and three capfuls at noon, and was disoriented in the afternoon and "woozy" after 15 minutes. The face was dull, and his vision was blurred. The same team of researchers confirmed that Gymnopilus validipes has Psilocybin (0.12 percentage) throughout the U.S. Three different species which include Gymnopilus spectabilis, have also been found to contain an alkaloid. Analyses of Gymnopilus spectabilis in the European Genus also yielded disappointing results. It was only through a sequence of circumstances that were unusual did the presence of psilocybin and its metabolites finally verified in Gymnopilus Genus European the fungus variety. Modern mushroom species was discovered growing on the root of a tree fern in Kew the botanical gardens of England from the beginning of May 1887 (also look at the page. 30 in the lower right). The findings led to the scientific publication of these mushrooms as a brand new species known as Flammula purpurata Cooke & Massee. In this regard we would like to thank Mordecai Cooke (1825-1914) who was a mycologist of exceptional skill and experience who studied numerous species of genus, including Psilocybe semilanceata. Cooke was among the very first person to develop a hypothesis about the blueing effect and to highlight its importance in the physiological sense (see the article on page. 16.). He identified Inocybe haemacta, as well as many other species of Panaeolus and was the first to identify the species mentioned above. Most interestingly, one of his first works included a compilation of folk tales , dubbed "The Seven Sisters Of Sleep" (1860) that was a narcotic plant inter-disciplinary research. Did he study a psychotropic mushroom maybe? We're certainly not likely to find the solution. In the end, the species known as Flammula was recognized as being indigenous and endemic to Australia as well as South America (Chile), in which the mushrooms blossom upon dead trees through May. The name of the mushroom was later altered into Gymnopilus purpuratus (Cooke and Massee) Sing. It was in 1983 that a large mushroom was discovered growing on the discarded wood chips and bark inside the Ribnitz particleboard plant Damgarten, located on the East German seaboard. It was initially classified as Tricholomopsis Rutilans (Schaeff. : Fr.) Sing. The magnificent and stunning mushroom was found to spore with dust-colored orange to rusty brown as well as a well-formed, translucent yellow cortina. It also changed color with pressure and it was erasing. Further research revealed that the fungus was from this species Gymnopilus purpuratus. It was a mushroom which was then cultivated in Europe after 100 years. Mixing liquid manure from pigs with leftover wood chips has created the necessary microclimate to promote the growth of mushrooms. A robust composting cycle gains from the dumping of liquid manure in heaps that are up to 20 yards in length and many yards high. The cycle must eliminate all types of waste. The temperatures within the scales were approximately 176 deg Fahrenheit. The Gymnopilus species was in a position to live in the top layer of the heaps together with others Asian or South American species with warm climates. It's not difficult to figure out precisely how Gymnopilus species came to Europe. In the latter part of the 1970s, Argentina brought in huge amounts of feed grains. So, some mushroom spores could have bonded to the grain and moved unharmed in the guts of porkers and then populated piles of compost. Because that the heaps in compost is cleared at every two years and used to fertilize nearby fields after two years after storage, the mushroom tend to sprout in new locations on stacks of wood as the spores spread (see figure 30, page. 40). But, due to changes in economic conditions and a growing ecological awareness within Eastern Germany, this composting process may be halted so that this species of mushroom disappears once more in Europe.

Conocybe Cyanopus tiny Mushrooms With a Potentity That is Amazing

The study of Mexico's magical mushrooms during the 50s R. Heim described the Conocybe species that was discovered in the 1950s. Conocybe siligineodes Heim was thought to be up to 8 centimeters (3.25 inches.) in length, and was a beautiful dark-orange-reddish-brown fungus that thrived on decaying wood, and was utilized by Indians for its psychotropic fungus. The species was not mentioned in the literature however, nor was the chemical compositions or findings of these specimens published. After years of fieldwork throughout Mexico, Guzman couldn't find the goat. Also, he can't find any possibility of using Conocybe specimens.

The description of Heim's brought about curiosity about the species' chemical composition. In earlier literature, 55 European species that were saprophytic were reduced to shadow life. In addition, distinguishing the species can be a challenge. The mushrooms are usually tiny and fragile, quickly disintegrating and showing up in mossy or grassy areas, which is where they can be often overlooked. In the year 1930 J. Schaffer found many Conocybe species growing rapidly in a fertilized grassy region close to Potsdam. Incredulous by the variety of colors and forms of the fungi and their colors, he decided to conduct the type of taxonomic classification that is required for studies on fungi. One plant he discovered within Potsdam, Berlin, and the Harz Mountains in Germany showed blue-colored discoloration on the bottom of its roots. Kuhner referred to the "Galera" plant under the name

Conocybecyanopoda within his 1934 Conocybe Genus monograph. The literature now calls this species Conocybecyanopus (Atk.) Kuhn. This blue-colored fungus was found within the U.S. (Ithaca, NY) in 1918, and was considered to be in competition in comparison to European mushroom species by the scientist Kuhner. This is a sufficient description of Conocybecyanopus since its blueish discoloration is an easily identifiable characteristic that differentiates the type of organism from others in Europe. Conocybe organisms. Cap: 0.3-2.5 cm long, roughly hemisphere-to-convex, striated, ocher to dark brown without grey-green stains. Stem: 2-4 cm long, 1-1,4 cm thick, whitish at first, slightly curved at the core, silvery later, stains bluish-green-especially at the base-in response to injury or age. Spores: 7-10x 5-4 um Basidia: four-spored, without cheilocystidia present, 18-25x6 5- 10, um Habitat woodlands or grassy areas, autumn to summer. The Conocybe Genus is part of the Bolbitiaceae family, which is similar to Coprinaceae family, which is a group of dark-spored fungi that form that Panaeolus group. Conocybe species are rare in Europe. The mushrooms are rarely seen in European list of discoveries. In addition to Schaffer's discovery the mushroom was reported to have been identified or described just twice!) (in the ex- East Germany territory over the last 60 years (both discovery took place in the 80s).

Yet, because of its lack of beauty it is a rare mycologist to are specialized in mycological studies of the Conocybe group. While the species is scarce, I might include a Conocybe cyanopus image within this publication (see Illustration 36 at. 56). 1 A clean Conocybe cyanopus specimen was very fortunate in terms of an analysis of the chemicals (see Table 9 at on p. 56). Psilocybin was first identified during a test of the Conocybe cyanopus fruiting body that were collected in September 4th, 1961 at Seattle, WA. There was no psilocin in the sample, but it is still unclear what they could be. Repke and his team of researchers have revealed the existence of baeocystin as well as psilocybin within U.S. and Canadian Conocybe community in 1977. The results were surprisingly, showing that there was no Psilocin. In 1982/83, Norwegian researchers verified the existence of small amounts of psilocybin, in addition to 0.330.55 percent of psilocybin an alkaloid that was also present on Finnish samples. In addition, Beug and Bigwood reported 0.93 percent of psilocybin found in Northwestern United States samples. It is interesting to note that the second specimen ever found within Eastern Germany was noticed on July 2, 1989 close to Potsdam near the city of Potsdam, where a number of Conocybe Cyanopus fruiting body grew in a sandy grassy area. The area that Schaffer was the first to contain the organisms more than 60 years ago is outside Potsdam city limits, and its precise location cannot more be identified. The research conducted in 1989 comprised five mushrooms that had levels of baeocystin and psilocybin comparable to those in Psilocybe semilanceata. Psilocybin levels were quite similar to those that were found in samples from The Northwestern United States. Spores of an of the plants that produce fruit developed on malt agar over some days, and then continued to grow very slowly in their permanent form or "sclerotia" in comparison with other species. The sclerotia did not show blue discoloration, and was it was found to have 0.25 percent psilocybin after drying and there was no evidence of other alkaloids. In conclusion, it's reasonable to believe that due to its tiny size and its extreme rarity the Conocybe cyanopus species isn't an important factor in European poisoning and neither will it likely to achieve recognition in the future. My analyses of other non-bluing Conocybe species like Conocybe Tenera (Schaeff. : Fr.) Fayod along with Conocybelactea (Lge) Metrod reported the presence of physiological inactive ingredients. A few Conocybe species samples from warmer countries haven't yet been tested, but they could provide remarkable chemical composition as well as alkaloid content tests.

Pluteus Salicinus: little-known wood-inhabiting Species

The Pluteaceae family comprises around the 45 European Pluteus species, some of which produce Psilocybin. In the past the Pluteus species belonged to the Amanitaceae family, which comprised"death mask" and its descendants "death mask" and its relatives along with an agaric fly both belonging to the Amanita group. Contrary to other psychoactive mushrooms discussed within this post, Pluteus is classified under light-spored mushrooms because of the spores' rose-colored color.

The literature has not yet reported accidental intoxications that affect Pluteus species. Saupe has provided the first lab evidence for the presence Psilocin and psilocin in the year 1981, when he examined Pluteus salicinus extracts (Pers. : Fr.) Kumm. In Illinois. It was interesting to note that psilocin was the alkaloid that had the highest concentration in the tests. This species of mushroom was discovered in Europe about two hundred years back. Since then, it has been hardly discussed in the literature, and only briefly, if frequently used taxonomic classification techniques are still confusing the species. Ricken (1915) identified the mushroom Pluteus petasatus. In expanding the classification of 1962 the following characteristics are a hallmark of Pluteus salicinus: medium-sized, rounded mushroom with more or less a deep blueish to bluish-green coloration. Older mushrooms can be olive-green. Caps that can be up to 8cm in diameter can be found in certain cases with edges that are lighter in color with a silver-gray appearance, and are rough and felt-like. They can be even more hairy and felt-like in at the center of your mouth. They are usually smooth and scaly. Stems that can reach 10 cm long, with unintentional gray-blue or gray-green discoloration near the base and a heightened color as they respond to pressure. The class also includes white mushrooms. These albino fruiting bodies are characterized by stems that exhibit a subtle grey-green coloration and their caps ' apex zones. Pluteus salicinus was recognized as "particularly unusual" to "not unusual" in Europe's forests of wet deciduous. Pluteus species are the last wood-destroying species, i.e. they develop saprophytically upon wood which appears discoloring and decaying because of the presence of various other species over many years. Pluteus salicinus is a fruiting species that grows between May and October on willow stumps lime trees, alder trees poplars, beech trees as well as maple trees, and possibly on wood remains from other species of trees too It is believed that this mushroom hasn't caused any harm can be confirmed through the visible appearance of their fruiting bodies on stumps of trees as individual mushrooms or in groups of a few. Pluteus salicinus is not as popular as other wood-living mushrooms. In a bizarre way, Kreisel has classified every Pluteus varieties to be "non-poisonous" within his 1987 handbook on mushrooms however the psilocybin (0.35 percent in dried mushrooms) was found in specimens from this genus in the year 2001 (North North America) as well as 1985 (Norway). There are instances of it within mushrooms of Holland, Finland, Sweden as well as France. However, the studies on France and Holland were all limited to a small fruiting bodies. While Stijve observed an average 0.25 percent psilocybin out of 20 samples taken in Switzerland between 1984 and 1986, dried mushrooms my analysis of non-bluing) (mushrooms collected from Thuringen, Germany in 1986 produced much higher levels of alkaloid.

Chapter 4: How To Remove The Poisonous

Substances

The majority of the fatal cases reported in the studies related to psychedelic mushroom usage involve the simultaneous usage of other drugs such as alcohol, in particular. Most likely the primary cause of hospital admissions that result from the use of psychedelics are "poor excursions" also known as "panic reactions", in which the individuals affected are extremely nervous or upset, disoriented or confused. Self-injury, accidents or attempts at suicide could result from intense psychotic experiences. Although there is no evidence linking Psilocybin with birth defects pregnant women should steer clear of the use of this drug.

Toxicity

Large psilocybin-related toxic effects. For mice, the median of lethal dosage (LD50) is 280 milligrams for each kilogram (mg/kg) roughly one-and-a-half times higher than caffeine. If administered intravenously to rabbits, LD50 is about 12.5 mg/kg. Psilocybin is approximately 1% of the total weight Psilocybecubensis mushrooms, thereby requiring or 1.7 kilograms (3.7 lbs) of dry mushrooms or 17.4 kilograms (37 lbs) in fresh mushrooms in order to attain the 280 mg/kg benefit for rats. Based on research conducted in animals the lethal dose of psilocybin was calculated to be 6 grams, or 1000 times the amount in milligrams. According to the Chemical Substances Toxic Effects Register has psilocybin as a high healing index at 641 (higher numbers indicate an improved safety profile) as compared with 199 or 21 and 21, respectively. The toxic dose for psilocybin is unknown for therapeutic or recreational levels and has not been well-documented until 2011 there were just two reports that can be attributed to the ingestion of hallucinogenic fungi (without any subsequent consumption of other substances) were reported in the scientific literature . These reports could refer to causes other than the psilocybin.

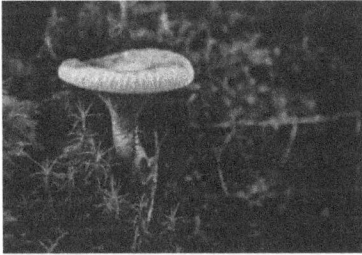

Mushroom Identification Make sure you avoid the most dangerous mistakes

Three teenagers looking to find psychoactive mushrooms in Whidbey Island, WA (USA) collected the organisms of Galerina animal on December 16 1981, fumbling that the mushrooms were part of an Psilocybe species. The three teens all fell sick after inhaling the mushrooms but did not declare their symptoms or consult a doctor for the next two days, putting themselves at risk of being charged with using the drug psilocybin. Two teens recovered fully following surgical treatment. The third victim passed away on the 24th of December 1981. According to Beug Bigwood and Bigwood the tragic incident underscores the dangers inherent to uninformed or incorrect identification of species of mushrooms, particularly when over-zealous regulatory and punitive actions can exacerbate a situation. Psilocybin-producing species and edible varieties of mushrooms, often have a common trait with different species. People who are casual about hunting for mushrooms and those who do not know how to are at risk of misconceptions that can result in accidental intoxications. The previous chapters provided examples of such unintentional intoxications. Absolutely, mycological keys of the present can be useful when deciding the genus and family of a mushroom sample that is not known. Yet, deciphering the particular species of fungi in problematic specimens can be extremely difficult, especially when the specimen falls into the general class that includes "LBMs" as well as "small mushroom species that are brown." We have only a few details about the Genus "LBM," as their habitats and variations in habitus aren't thoroughly studied. Unexpectedly, the reference literature is often stifled by inadequate descriptions that fail to consider the most important criteria to distinguish distinct species from other species. I can recall my first efforts to determine foreign species using specific descriptions from traditional mycological research books. I see some of the characteristics mentioned as describing a variety of species, often with very specific descriptions. When I compared my specimens against the source document I noticed a tendency to overlook some of the more intricate specifics, however "my mushrooms" will better fit the explanations. Naturally, it led to errors. Fortunately, once I contacted fellow mycologist colleagues, I could soon discover mistakes and correct them. According to my experience, abilities to recognize mushrooms and the associated competence are honed over time through extensive fieldwork, consultation with mycological experts in the field as well as a thorough study of the sample of the information in poor references. The literature suggests that Psilocybe semilanceata is a species that is easily identified at prime spots using the diagnostic tools. Psilocybe semilanceata is renowned for its distinct appearance and appearance, which is why microscopic tests are not required to differentiate this fungus from other grass-dwelling species. The problem is for

Psilocybe species is different, however, thrives on wood waste, is depicted by the tragic tale at the start of the book. As compared to Europe and the European continent, this North American mycoflora includes, in the beginning an even more extensive and varied range of species. Avert yourself from toxic amatoxins! Galerina produces a variety of toxic mushrooms. The species is harmful because they contain the same lethal amatoxins that are found in"the "death cap" (Amanita phalloides) as well as its cousins of"death angel" and "death angel" and the "death angel." The toxins they produce are pervasive and without symptoms for approximately 12 hours. In this time frame pollutants can cause significant permanent internal damage. This is the reason why, once diagnosed some cases can be fatal. The most well-known North American species is Galerinaautumnalis (Peck) Singer & Smith as well as other Psilocybe species, thrives on wood waste in forests and parks. On first sight, Galerinaautumnalis resembles Psilocybestuntzii Guzman & Ott in the same location, both species can be found side-by-side. Galerina however, will not change into blue. I have once stumbled across an uncultivated field with the set of Psilocybestuntzii specimens wrapped in the Galerina leaf.

The mushrooms were so interspersed that only spore analysis could discern distinct fruiting bodies. Pholiotinafilaris Song. Is there a second North American animal known to contain amatoxins? In the same way, these toxins were not found in these animals' European samples. Pholiotinafilaris (Fr.) Perform. It is likely that there are different species that is found on both continents. At least, an European Galerina organisms (Galerinamarginata (Fr.) Kuhn.) produces the same toxins that are found in the mushroom "death caps." The organism is able to grow in the wood substrates that are decreasing and is comprised of approximately one-third of amanitins within Amanita phalloides. Incredibly, older mushroom books mention Galerinamarginata as edible. In the previous chapter about the species Panaeolus I discussed the ability to spot problems that can be linked to the agricultural zones "invaded" by non-native species. Because of their rapid growth, Panaeolus species can often produce fruit in artificially-cultivated zones long before the cultivating species develop there. Chapter 3.3 explains the 1970 toxicity incident involving the Leipzig-based Panaeolussubbalteatus. In that scenario, the intruding species was confused for Strophariarugoso-annulata Farlow, based on information from a mushroom journal. No one noticed the obvious difference between the text from the publication and actual features, excluding it being possible that tiny amount of samples suggested that the mushrooms hadn't grown as large as they were in the book claims. This false hypothesis reveals the misperceptions of amateurs who believe that they're experts. For instance certain mycophiles have proved to be convinced that they will be able to identify these species later in coming years. That's why one particular mushroom hunter ate Inocybeaeruginascens spores that he thought could be ring-shaped mushrooms. In a similar case of Inocybeaeruginascens intoxication, mushrooms were selected as white champignons, although this common culinary mushroom does not resemble Inocybeaeruginascens, either in size or shape. In the end, these tragic events also contributed to the discovery of biochemistry in mushrooms. In this particular instance I'd like to emphasize that Inocybes hallucinogenic species could easily be confused with the extremely toxic Inocybe species that have mucarine. In his Psilocybe Genus research, Guzman observed a common characteristic of hallucinogenic species, as well as the bluing reaction, which is the smell or taste of flour. In addition to the inherent subjective nature of our senses of smell and taste an odor that is commonplace is not a characteristic of European species.

Chapter 5: Benefits In Personal Development

When autumn transforms into winter, it is when a lot of travelers head for the more remote parts of the country to wander for hours around the area. Their love object is the mysterious, small creatures known as "Liberty Cap,"" the hallucinogen that is naturally found in the UK. Magic mushrooms are widely distributed and nearly every culture has a long-standing, religious connection to these vital drugs. There is evidence in stone carvings, for example that North African aboriginal Saharan tribes could have been using mushrooms since approximately 9000 BC. In the UK present, the magical season of foraging for mushrooms has increased from around 33 autumn days of fruiting, to more than 70 because of the changing climate. Professor. Lynne Boddy, a fungal ecologist, says, "Climate change has had profound effects on the time of the year that fruiting occurs and every year, the season's end and start times are based on temperature. However, we can observe that it was mostly constant until the end of the 1970s. In general, however the first date for fruiting is also significantly earlier in the year than it was before and the last one is later." A lot of people hunt them for the pleasure of the after-consumption euphoria outcomes. Some people make use of the fungus to gain spiritual wisdom and knowledge. The irony is that new research has confirmed the legends of health benefits from eating magical mushrooms.

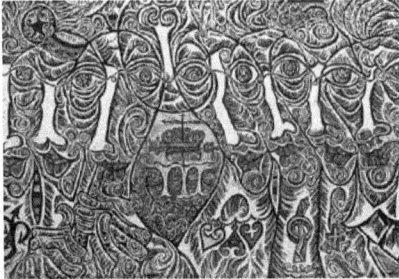

1. Increase in "Openness" as well as other beneficial Changes in Personality

We are all born with an open and compassionate, eager to connect, grow and grow into sentient beings. Events that may cause suffering and hinder us from living our lives. Examples of obvious ones include broken hearts. may not be as inclined to romantic future opportunities. Anyone who has a history of negative experiences relating to life problems will shut down to limit new experiences. It's definitely helpful when this data can help us however, in many instances we may shut down more than we really need to and limit our potential through limiting opportunities and experiences that are new. Psilocybin could be helpful in these situations. Researchers have found "significant increase in transparency after an intense psilocybin dose" in a study from 2011. Transparency is a term used in psychology to describe someone's willingness to accept new experiences. It is associated with traits such as creativity creative thinking, creativity, and pleasure. Transparency generally increases during an psilocybin-related session, but was much above the baseline for over a year after the event in around 60% of the participants. The law does not prohibit psychedelics since a compassionate government is worried that you may jump out of an unintentional third-story window. They are prohibited due to their impact on the awareness system and social attitudes and the structures of information processing. They offer the possibility that what you think you know isn't true.

Two-Smoking, Other Drugs and Addictions

If you're experiencing negative behaviors that are causing you to be unhappy the psychedelics can change your life. They have also been proven to treat addiction-causing substances like nicotine and cocaine. In 2008 the Beckley Foundation's Amanda Feilding launched a partnership with Johns Hopkins University on a pilot study that explored psychotherapy to fight nicotine addiction. A continued support from the Heffter Research Institute is in support of the psilocybin study as a possible treatment for addiction disorders caused by substances.

3. Reduce Depression

Psilocybin is the active ingredient of the psychoactive mushroom, given many great civilizations' philosophical and cultural base. The Aztecs referred to teonanacatl as' divine mushroom,' and modern neuroscience has shown how psilocybin combines in the brain with serotonin receptors to create a variety of consciousness-altering results. Recent research has shown how effective magical mushrooms can be used to combat depression. In some instances, a single dose could help alleviate symptoms for life.

4. Let go of your Ego and increase Creativity

Psilocybin, a psychoactive drug in general, and psychedel specifically, can produce states in which our conscious perception of the world is freed from our ego, which may be exposed as a false concept. If used in the right context according to a report from 2017 that a temporary depletion of the ego can be beneficial. These massive, sometimes life-altering experiences allow us to feel incredibly in touch and alive. They also encourage creativity.

5. How magic Mushrooms can improve mental health

Although magic mushrooms are generally disregarded and often seen as risky "party substances," they are presented in a more positive way by an organization that studies them. They are not only more secure than most people think and have a huge potential to aid in various mental health issues. According to neuroscientist Nick Jikomes notes for a Harvard science journal, psychedelics generally contain "negligible possibility of creating a habit." Some psychedelics could aid in the treatment of addictions to addictive drugs like nicotine and cocaine. Magic mushrooms are gradually being regarded as a wonder drug that can be used for therapeutic purposes. Research has demonstrated positive effects for depression, like an investigation in 2017 that revealed the psilocybin "may efficiently restore the activity of major brain circuits that are believed to play a part during depression." The substance is believed to increase your brain's emotional responsiveness an additional study has found which suggests it could help relieve depression , without the "emotional dulling" that is often associated with the traditional. Psilocybin can provide a profound release from anxiety for people suffering from life-threatening cancer. One study showed that low doses psilocybin-in conjunction with psychotherapy- helped cancer patients conquer their depression and anxiety related to diagnosis and lead to a lasting improvement in their quality of life and happiness. Six months after the initial dose (which was only four to six hours) around 80percent of patients showed significant reductions in depression and anxiety. 83% reported greater happiness in their lives. The majority of respondents rated their psilocybin treatment as one of their five most memorable experiences in their lives. Despite the growing interest in research, the traditional magical mushroom caricatures appear to be changing quickly. As an example, Denver and Oakland's U.S. populations were decriminalized in 2019 and similar initiatives are being implemented across the nation as well as at the state levels. Recently, psilocybin was advertised as the "breakthrough treatment" that could help with U.S. depressive. A large study in the latter part of 2019 found "no negative effects that were serious" in healthy volunteers and no negative impact on the emotional or cognitive functions. In addition, with the growing interest and enthusiasm for the science of psilocybin, we might be closer to the edge of understanding. In the year 2019 Johns Hopkins University announced the establishment of the one-of-a-kind $17 million Center for Psychedelic and Consciousness Research which was the first study center within the U.S. and the world's largest. "The center's establishment marks an exciting new era in the field of psychological and therapeutic science by examining this unique and fascinating category of pharmacological compounds," stated the director Roland Griffiths, a professor of behavioral biology at Johns Hopkins.

Chapter 6: Step By Step Cultivation Process

Magic mushrooms are among the most simple plants to cultivate. They need particular parameters and patience. The kits that a lot of online stores offer include a perlite and vermiculite base that contains mycelium, that's where shrooms originate from. The process of activating and cultivating your own shrooms is a breeze, continue going for the complete instruction on how to do it correctly. Every variety of mushroom has distinct features due to the fact that they are from diverse regions of the globe.

Certain varieties are more easy to cultivate than others, while some are more robust and some produce more than others. They tend to grow in a variety of forms that you can observe when they are launched. The photo below shows one particular strain, often called 'Cambodian' and predicted to grow the same day. The Cambodian shrooms produced hardly any mycelium, but the larger ones are much more rapid. If you've never had the chance to grow magical mushrooms before, then we suggest an alternative called Mexican. The specific strain is able to adapt more easily to humidity and temperature and, therefore, even if you don't provide the ideal conditions, it has the chance to be successful.

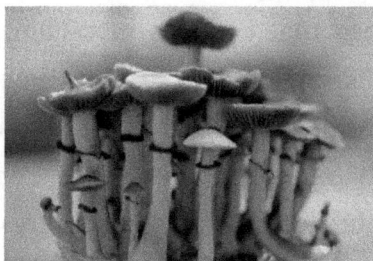

The Basic Parameters for Magic Mushrooms

Lighting

One of the major aspects of growing magical mushroom is how much light they receive and their quality. They cannot be supplied with directly lit. They can be created with sunlight or a standard light bulb but not in the form of a substrate. In terms of the amount of light required is concerned, it can be challenging, as mushrooms naturally grow in the open forests, spending a good amount of their time at evening. If you are cultivating them in light, the only thing you have to do is open the curtains and place the mushrooms in the opposite end of your window, and make sure that they aren't directly exposed to sunlight. If you're using light sources within your home it is necessary to place it so that it doesn't reflect directly on the ground.

Humidity

Humidity is crucial since it triggers the mycelium that makes shrooms grow. To ensure the proper humidity, you can use the tiny greenhouse propagator. Filter the substratum to hydrate it or osmosis vapor. Never make use of tap water. When you add waterto the container, the substratum will expand, which is why you'll need to gradually move it around to ensure it's evenly filled with water. When it's fully saturated, remove any water left-if it's not removed from the base of the container, it could cause the growth of fungi. Most mushroom kits come with a bag that you can make into a propagator however, if you're looking for the best results , we recommend getting a greenhouse-specific propagator. In order to trigger mycelium, you have to keep the humidity within the propagator at 90 percent for at least two days. This means that you'll have to add water to the bottom of your propagator, not the container for your substrate. The water can also be filtering or osmosis. Another method is to ensure that the cover stays over the tubing, this will create the humidity. It is necessary to reduce humidity to around 70% within the first two days. This is simple to achieve by fiddling around with the tiny windows that are on the sides of your propagator.

Temperature:

Temperature is an additional crucial aspect; mushrooms generally develop in between the 21st and 24th degrees C So if you're looking to grow the most amount of mushrooms as you can We suggest you place your propagator at the center. If you're intending to plant them cold then you could always purchase an insulated propagator or a heated blanket to cover the propagator. If you cultivate your mushrooms at temperatures below 21 degrees C the mushrooms are likely to grow slower and produce less mushrooms once the mycelium has been filled the mycelium has only enough time to grow mushrooms.

Hygiene:

The last but not last, the rising magical mushrooms require cleanliness and a tidy environment. They are extremely sensitive and require a clean and sterilized space. Don't be touching them with your fingers and use gloves made of latex when handling the box , and in the event that you have to, put on a face mask. Try to avoid changing the surroundings around them as much as you can. Don't drink, apply deodorant or any other chemical sprays in the room they're in, or they could become polluted and fail to grow correctly. Your magic mushroom kits will have the proper temperatures, humidity, lighting and a clean environment that will produce many eye-catching psychedelic visions. Many online stores offer everything you require to grow your magical mushrooms, right from the kits themselves , to things such as heated mats, thermo-hygrometers and even complete scientific research kit.

Harvesting

In 7-14 days, you'll begin to see the first few mushrooms emerge. In the next few days they'll appear all over the place. If you examine them at least once a day, you'll likely observe them growing just a few centimeters each day. They'll likely be ready after approximately 3-4 days, but you'll need to allow them to dry for a few more days before you are able to consume the mushrooms. Make sure you wear gloves before removing the mushrooms. Then, apply pressure to them using your fingers and squeeze them with your fingertips. The mushrooms will see them come out naturally. They're quite sensitive and if you touch them, they'll turn to a dark hue for a couple of hours. It's normal, don't fret about decay or waste as they're edible. If you remove each and every mushroom do not discard the bottle. Mycelium in bottles can be active for quite a while dependent on the environment. After a few days you could be able to have a new harvest of mushrooms. If you have perfect conditions it is possible to get three or four mushrooms out of a single container.

How to grow Magic Mushrooms in Seven Steps

Equipment

* 12 wide mouth half-pint containers that have lids (make sure you get a wide mouth)

* Cup to measure

* Small nail and hammer

Large mixing bowl, as well as spoon

* Strainer

* Tinfoil (heavy-duty)

* Large pot for cooking with a lid that is tight (or the Instant Pot)

* Small towel

* Microspore tape

Storage box made of clear plastic 50-115 L

* 1/4 inch drill bit/Drill

* Perlite

* Mist spray bottle

* Ingredients

Spore Syringe: 10-12 cc

The organic brown rice can also be called brown rice flour (use the coffee grinder for brown rice)

* Vermiculite, medium/fine

* Bottled water for consumption (preferably distilled)

* Sanitation Items

* 70 70% Isopropyl alcohol as well as Lysol (or equivalent)

*BIC lighter (or propane torch)

* Air sanitizer

• Latex glove, surgical mask and a glove box (optional)

The Process

Once you've bought all the necessary ingredients, it's time to begin the process of cultivation at home. We've broken down the process of growing psychedelic mushrooms in six steps:

Step 1: Preparation

Step 2: Innoculation

3. Colonization

Step 4 Preparing the chamber for growing

* Step 5: Fruiting

* Step 6: Harvesting

* Step 7 Storage and drying

Step 1. Preparation

Clean the jars using alcohol to remove any traces of bacteria. Then employ a nail and hammer to make four holes into the lids, in a uniform spacing.

* Then make the substrate ready by mixing 2/3 cup vermiculite with 1/4 cup water into the bowl of mixing.

• Cleanse the strainer by using alcohol, and then remove any excess water from the mixture.

* Add the 1/4 cup of brown rice flour per half-pint container (meaning three cups twelve jars) to the bowl , then blend with the moist vermiculite.

Following that, you need filling the jars up to within a half-inch of the edge.

* Be careful not to pack too tight. Be sure to clean the upper inch with alcohol.

* Finish off the containers with a layer of dry vermiculite.

It's now time to steam sterilize the jars. Screw the lids securely and cover the jars with aluminum foil.

* Secure your foil's edges with the sides to keep condensation from leaking through.

* Place the towel into the pot , then put the jars on top. This will stop water from splashing , and could lead to entering the substrate.

Add tap water to the degree halfway across the sides. Then, bring to a simmer with the jars still standing upright. Put the lid on tightly and steam for about 75 to 90 minutes.

• A pressure cooker (or Instant Pot) that is set to run for sixty minutes and 15 PSI is also a good option.

After the steaming has finished, put the containers inside the pot a few hours. They should be kept at room temperature before you begin the inoculation process.

Step 2: Innoculation

The best method of inoculating is to use an airbox. First, clean the entire area, and then use gloves made of latex. If you do not have an airbox, it's acceptable, but increases the risk of contamination.

Cleanse and making the needle. Utilize a lighter to warm the entire length of the syringe needle until it's hot red.

* Let it cool, then wipe it with alcohol and don't touch it with your fingers.

* Pull the plunger back as well as shake the syringe in order to evenly disperse the spores.

Remove the foil from the jars, and then insert the syringe so as it can pass in one of the holes.

* Pour approximately 1/4 cup of the solution of spores into the sides of the jar, but not directly onto the surface.

Repeat for each hole by wiping the needle clean with alcohol in between each.

Cover the holes using microspore tape, then set the jar aside, taking the foil cut off.

Step 3. Colonization

In the past, you've put in many hours of work to make the psychoactive mushrooms. Now, the process becomes more of a waiting game.

* Make sure to keep the jars clear of debris and away from the way (a crawl space or basement may be ideal).

Do not expose yourself to direct light and avoid temperatures between 70-80 degrees F (room temperature).

Between 7 and 14 days, you will begin to see white, fluffy mycelium.

If you notice any unusual smells or colors remove the jars immediately.

Certain chemicals are dangerous for humans, in spite of the debate on the internet suggests.

* After 3 to 4 weeks, you will have at minimum 6 jars that are successful.

* Allow an additional seven days for the mycelium to build up the grip to the surface.

* Be aware that some grow kits are able to be completed in as little as the span of 21 days (3 weeks) thus those tools might be more efficient.

4. Preparing your grow chamber

* Open the storage container made of plastic and drill 1/4-inch holes 2 inches apart on the sides, base and the lid.

* Inject hole from inside to prevent cracking.

* Place the box on top of four solid objects in order so that airflow can flow beneath it.

* Cover the underside of the box to stop the possibility of moisture loss.

* Pour perlite into an aerator and run it under cold tap water until it begins to soak.

* After the perlite has been drained put it in the base in the chamber.

Repeat until you have an additional layer of perlite that is about 4-5 inches in depth.

Step 5: Fruiting

Then, open the jars and take off the vermiculite layer that is dry. The process will result in tiny"cakes" of white "cakes". If they don't come out, simply tap the bottle gently until the cake is released onto the surface that has been disinfected.

* Wash the cakes, place them in the container of plastic filled with water and then submerge them under the surface (so they're completely covered).

It's easy to pour the water into an empty plastic container, fill it with water, then place another container of plastic to the top of the jars so that they stay submerged.

* Store them for about 24 hours, so they can rehydrate.

* Roll the White cakes with vermiculite. Then, you'll add dry vermiculite, then roll the cakes to coat them evenly, and it will help retain the moisture.

* Cut a square of tin foil per cake (ensuring it is not touching the surface of perlite) and then arrange your cakes over top equally spaced within the chamber.

Spray the cakes with the bottle and then blow the lid prior to closing it.

* Utilizing the spray bottle, spray at least four times per day to ensure that the humidity remains.

* Don't soak the.e cakes in water, but.

* Make sure to blow the lid up to six times per day in order to improve the flow of air.

Step 6: Harvesting

The last step is to remove the bodies that are fruiting from the growing. They will be visible in the form of bumps, and then pins. In about 10 to 14 days, they'll be ready to be harvested.

Once you're ready, pick the mushrooms near the cake. As they get closer to maturity, their strength diminishes. Pick them earlier for harvesting.

Step 7 7. Drying and storage

Dry mushrooms are still moist that can result in the rotting of. Psilocybin mushrooms could last just several weeks. There are many methods to dehydrate these magical mushrooms. The easiest is to lay them on a piece of paper before the fan, but it will leave moisture. The most effective method is to make use of a dehydrator. this is the method we suggest.

Step 8: Continue to Grow Shrooms and Again

When you've completed all the steps, be proud! You're an excellent person for taking it one step at a. The process of learning how to grow the psychedelic mushrooms won't be over but. It's possible to continue. The cake you gathered can be used again. One method to reuse them is to dry them for after a couple of days, and then follow this "dunking" technique (without using vermiculite). Return them to the grow chamber with mist as well as a fan. After that, you'll be able to have one or two (if there are not two) batch of psilocybin mushrooms.

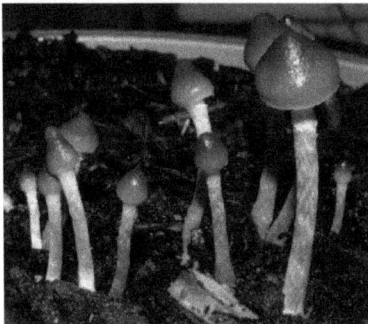

Chapter 7: Tips To Take Magic Mushrooms

For a long time magical mushrooms were utilized to produce experiences that ranged from euphoria and mystical sensations. For beginners, it is best to prepare for this experience and there are some rules of thumb to make sure that you will want to go back for your initial experience and any subsequent ones. The experience of having magical Mushrooms is unique to any other. In certain communities they've been utilized for centuries to promote spiritual experiences and to feel connected to the spiritual realm.

As with any substance that is psychoactive, taking your time taking a close look at the sensation is crucial. According to Timothy Leary said, "location and the atmosphere" is a significant factor to do with the experience of shrooms. Here are some helpful suggestions for professionals about what to do and how to think about when working with Psilocybin.

Feel Good To Start Tripping

The effects of mushrooms can alter moods and the affect your mood when you experience these. If you're not feeling good or unhappy, you're more likely to have a difficult experience. Be in a more positive and A Trustworthy Atmosphere in a relaxed space with those you know. An unsatisfactory or "solid" excursion in a foreign setting can lead to an unsatisfactory experience. It is also advised for novices to truffles and novices to bring an "sitter" accompanying you on the entire journey. Sitting with a sitter means a responsible person who makes sure everything runs smoothly and assists you and other travelers on the journey to have a good time.

Make Yourself

Prepare your for coffee, fruit juice teas, herbal teas, and some light snacks. Magic truffles last between three to six hours. In this time it is fine to eat something however you might feel hungry. It is also possible to find your route to the refrigerator challenging and you should have food on hand.

Take a trip to the Magic Mushrooms on an Unfulfilled Stomach

Drink nothing for at most three hours prior to taking shrooms. This means that the psilocybin is likely to be absorbed faster in your system. You're significantly less likely to be afflicted by the confusion that is often experienced in the initial stages of trips.

Avoid combining Shrooms with other mind-altering substances.

Drugs You shouldn't use magic mushrooms in conjunction with other substances that alter your mind. The magical experience of magic mushrooms differs from any experience you've experienced. Combining them with opioids can make for a disastrous trip. But, others have reported that taking a small amount of cannabis may help to ease the nausea some users are experiencing at the beginning of their trip. It also helps with the anxiety and anxiety. Make sure you're not professional shroom customer.

161

How many Magic Mushrooms will I need to take?

It's not a "can" regarding dosage. It's better to take it slow and be cautious. If you've never tried shrooms before and are still a beginner to truffles, you might not know the degree of your sensitivity to the psilocybin. Be aware that the doses of truffles vary from those of a mushroom. In any case, you must attain any thresholds. One quarter of one gram dried shrooms is commonly referred to as to be the "threshold dosage," ensuring a patient gets a pleasant experience but not really notice any outcomes. Also bright colors and bright lighting can give an "starry" appearance however they are not that much. The pupils may dilate, there is a possibility of some dizziness, or you could be able to have "hallucinations" near some of the peripheral edges.

A "normal" dose of 1-2.5gm is enough to create a genuine experience. Feel nausea. The eyes expand, and the heart rate and blood pressure increase (although it's not at a hazardous amount). Certain people still feel the sensation of "cooling" during the time the trip commences.

Sometimes, huge graphics appear, along with dream-like images of trips to shrooms. The emotions are also complex and distorted. Sitting with a friend is crucial, particularly for new users. A lot of negative emotions that can arise during this period are characterized by extreme self-doubt. In reality, many users talk about the "ego-loss" when they are in a positive setting as a very pleasant experience. It also refers to an unrestricted enjoyment of the universe without any purpose, worry or control.

Are Magic Mushrooms dangerous?

There isn't a single answer, but clearly there is no answer. The evidence for fatal overdoses is not extensive and psilocybin isn't considered hazardous. Most of the time, psilocybin doesn't cause you to lose sight of reality. You won't turn psychotic or go on a journey for the rest of your life. However, if you've got an established history of mental illness or a history of mental illness, it could exacerbate these symptoms. However, they are the most potent drug available to the majority of people.

How do you describe Good Like?

That's user-dependent. The colors of items are vibrant. Also, people feel happy being in awe. Sound waves echo, and you could not know if they took place. Additionally, you will be able to "cast" intricate geometric patterns while closing your eyes. Users also describe a "freedom" sensation. Thought trains are able to flow effortlessly and some shroom-trippers enjoy an "better view" about their lives. Many users experience "owing to gods" or are experiencing "many different aspects" of consciousness.

Chapter 8: Things You Would Like To Know

About A Room That Contain General Information

And The Statistics

As with all things, it's important to gather details. This section provides some basic information about psilocybin and also some facts and figures related to their use and psychedelic usage generally.

General information

One of the primary things you should be aware of about psilocybin is that they are not toxic or addicting. The most commonly held belief about them is that they are poisonous , and the poison can cause an euphoric feeling.

It is possible to say that this is the case however only if the chemicals are described as substances that cause the "intoxicated" condition or an altered state. If this is the case, then this definition includes any medication, which includes marijuana and caffeine as well as alcohol and nicotine. But, if your definition of poisonous includes anything that has a harmful impact on your body, then psilocybin mushroom don't belong in this category. They're less toxic than the other drugs listed with the exception of marijuana that has no harmful negative effects. Magic mushrooms do not cause serious health effects. According to another myth they do not cause bleeding in the stomach or brain. Also, they don't result in kidney damage. The report from 1981 showed no adverse effects from the consumption of mushrooms in healthy individuals, with the exception of eyes that are dilated and extremely sensitive reflexes when traveling. In addition, overdoses are unlikely , as the typical "heroic" or huge dose is around 5 grams in dried mushrooms. In order to reach the threshold for overdose you must consume approximately 1.7 tonnes of dried mushrooms. Let your body digest everything immediately. For Americans that's 3 pounds worth of dried mushrooms. It's a fact. take place. (For maths enthusiasts it's a sign that the system is being drained.

Mushrooms are 10 times more powerful than fresh mushrooms, based on weight. Another study indicates that the majority of COG information was originally obtained through water). While it is among the most illegal drugs, with no therapeutic uses and a significant abuse potential Psilocybin is a drug with a low possibility of abuse. It has been proven to be effective in treating addiction. Additionally, tolerance grows quickly when using psilocybin or other psychedelics. As such, it's difficult to use it for long periods of time. In the event that it raises doubts, the tolerance will decrease in a matter of days. The most common rule is that for psychedelics who are deciding to use for two days and the third day, they is required to eat twice in the morning to achieve the same effects. The planning of the trip is more efficient. This is especially true when you wish to extend the duration of your trip. Most of the time the process of taking in more hallucinogens following hitting the maximum dosage can result in the trip to be longer however it does not raise the intensity unless a larger dose is consumed. Before blindly adhering to this advice, keep in mind that every person's body chemistry is unique. In the case of psilocybin it's difficult to determine the exact dosage and therefore caution is advised. Another concern is that psilocybin or other psychedelic mushrooms can drive you insane. This is not the scenario. But, they do are arousing experience and experiences. If you are exploring hallucinogens for first time, it's essential to have a specialist guide to give you the foundation in the most intense times. It is also crucial to start small until you understand how your body and your mind will react to this sensation. If you've never had this before and are thinking about this possibility, ensure you travel with people who you like, with whom you have complete trust and with whom you feel secure. Be sure the atmosphere is well-controlled, for instance an inviting, peaceful and tidy space inside where you can lay down should you like or in a peaceful environment that allows you to relax and connect with the nature. It could be it's a good idea to take an excursion and attend an event or a club however if you don't have experience they aren't as enjoyable as you imagine they'll be. Discover how this might impact you in the beginning. It will be appreciated later. If you are immersed in hallucinogens such as psilocybin, or any other the one thing you'd like to keep in mind and maybe even remember is that you're not insane and are not going to be insane throughout the rest of your life. The road ahead will be upwards and downwards but you'll soon be back to normal. In the meantime, take a deep breath. If you've got something to do, let it come to you. Don't resist. Check out what they're showing you and save the images to come back future reference. It's not required to make major decisions in this area. It's to be done the future. There are two activities you should be doing.

It is important to be cautious when handling psilocybin mushroom. The first step is to be sure that any mushrooms you consume are psilocybin and not other species of similar nature. That means that you do not intend to hunt for mushrooms based upon the pictures within the text or the Internet. This applies to this book and any other. If you intend to gather mushrooms, work with a knowledgeable individual who's had experience collecting and consumed - mushrooms within the area you're looking to collect. Second, while mushrooms and other psychedelics aren't harmful, if you consume more than you're familiar with, you might make a mistake or even sensible in the moment however it appears to be. In other situations, I believe it was not an appropriate decision. A reliable guide or babysitter will ensure that this doesn't occur. Experience is also helpful and so is the selection of time. For instance, tripping when driving, or operating heavy machineryis not an ideal idea. It's not about jumping lines or seeing whether you've suddenly acquired abilities to glide or even roll. It's possible, but do a little research before you try this idea. The journey can start anywhere from 20 minutes up to an hour following consumption.

From now from now, the experience will take between four and six hours. It is recommended to set aside one day prior to the event to review your goals and reflect on your current situation. It is also suggested that you spend the day following the completion of what you've been through. This also allows you to relax before heading to work or any other unwelcome demands. Also, you'll frequently be told "bad traveling" scary stories. They're not necessarily the result of the substance in itself. They are more of a situation in which anxiety and other mental disorders become worse and allowed to progress. It is imperative to know that psilocybin is not to be utilized in cases of schizophrenia in the family or if you are suffering from a mental health issue. The drug may trigger psychotic episodes. When psilocybin is found to be utilized for therapeutic reasons in the context of post-traumatic stress or anxiety disorder, it is done under strict clinical conditions and under medical supervision. Don't attempt it on your own. If you're not experiencing these issues, just calm down and breathe it will all be perfectly. If you establish a routine of deep relaxation when traveling and are able to experience new thoughts and feelings and thoughts, you'll probably never have an "bad experience" in your lifetime regardless of how many times you've had the psychedelic sensation. It's all up to you. One of the most important things that psychedelics can provide us with is the ability to improve our feelings and thoughts. If you are able to accept the inner thoughts and feelings that are going on within you and accept it, you'll be perfectly fine. If you attempt to run away and distract yourself, or fall to sleep or, generally escape in any way, you'll see that it doesn't work. We will never be free of ourselves from. Finding ourselves in these situations with a sense of security can teach us how to relax and develop an inner sense of acceptance. The safe use of the technique will be explained in greater detail below.

Statistics and Data

Here are some facts and figures on psilocybin gathered from a range of studies. In an earlier survey 83% of respondents said that the experience they had with psilocybin was among the five most significant memories of their lives. In an investigation in which 94% of the people who had used psilocybin fungi reported that their event positively changed their lives.

A study piloted on the psilocybin plant in the lab of Johns Hopkins University suggests that the use of psilocybin could help in the fight against nicotine dependence. 89% of participants in another study scored positive or moderate improvements after a treatment using Psilocybin. These indicators remained consistent after a full year of monitoring. A study of magnetic resonance in 2014 regarding the effect of psilocybin the nervous system revealed the simultaneous activity of areas like the hippocampus and the anterior cortex, regions of the brain in which the activity is not coordinated with normal awakening awareness. Similar studies showed an incredibly dramatic shift in the way the brain where various parts of the brain communicated and synchronized above what is seen in normal brain activity. A study in 2011 that assessed the effects of psilocybin on five areas of personality that are crucial to us (neuroticism, extroversionand openness, kindness , and awareness) demonstrated that transparency grew significantly following the high-dose session and that the quality "remained far above the norm for more than a full year after having the treatment." Many claim that the experience of the effects of psilocybin cause the temporary dissolution of the self. A study from 2017 indicates that this brief dissolution of the ego can help in constructively rethinking our perception of the world. Additionally, those who have had this experience retain the ability to change their subjective viewpoint that is different from what we see in people who haven't experienced a psychedelic sensation. A different study revealed that mice who received psilocybin-based mushrooms are less likely to be frozen in extreme circumstances than those in the group that was in control. In light of these studies, researchers are studying the potential of psilocybin for the treatment of PTSD. In a study on drug rehabilitation facilities in central and western Europe hallucinogens were found to be the most commonly used drugs. They only accounted for 0.3 percent of requests for treatment. A study from 2016 found an average of 84% the people who had a psychedelic experience throughout their lives did it to better understand themselves 60 percent of people took psychedelics to increase their spiritual awareness and 36% to deal with issues. Emotional. Chapter 3. Effects of the pharmaceutical process and Psilocybin Pharmacology Biochemistry psychoedelic impacts (internal sensorial impressions) psychoedelic effects psychological effects of psychedelics

Chapter 9: Identification Of The Mushroom

The process of identifying mushrooms can be daunting and must be handled with caution. In this guide it will help you identify the most important functions needed for identifying mushrooms correctly. This guide can be used to make the list of things to record and check in the event that you encounter an unfamiliar species. Finding out about mushrooms can be an enjoyable way to increase your confidence and, with appropriate knowledge, will offer you the best food to eat.

1. Examine the date and time Find out what foods you could expect to see according to your location and the time. Find out which species of

mushrooms are found in your area of the globe; this can significantly narrow down the list of species that could be found. Be aware of the conditions. Some fungi occur only in a particular range (spring/summer/autumn/winter).

2. Find out how the fungus is able to grow organically: wooden floors. The leaves are composted is found in deciduous and sterile trees.

3. Identifies the species as well as the level of security once the mushroom is identified as a part of the u-tree species. Mycorrhizal bacteria may be parasites can be found or are related to. Mycorrhizal fungi can be found in tree roots and this system is at the root of trees that is far more extensive. It is often difficult to recognize, particularly when the amount that samples are taken decreases. These radial mycorrhizal mycorrhizal mushrooms are at the foundation of an rise in the sleeves. Mycorrhizal mushrooms can form fairytale-like circles that are connected with dead or living trees. Parasitic fungi spread in the lower part of the tree or within the woodland. Find out where you are and the mushrooms that

have been enlarged. Remember that fungal nets are able to live even after the plant dies.

4. Take note of the surrounding. Some species need specific development environments.

5. Analysis of poop, or reasons behind the type of cork being investigated. Also, think about the age that the mushrooms have reached. You: a convex? Hemispherical. Avoid using it only as half eggs. Conical: cone-shaped.

Umbonate: With a basic Umbi (curved bump) and an open lid. Umbilicate: having a round and straight slot, similar to the inside to an umbrella. Papillary With an acute tumor with a half-time amount. Funnel: a heartbreaking central sadness that forms tubes.
Sunk: dark hood with a wider margin towards the center.

Floor: flat roof. Cylindrical: rounded shirts with an extremely large perpendicularly curved hood (e.g. scalpy hair).

Support Restrictions on climbing on wood usually a spherical form: completely active. I just discovered that the balloons are inflated, and you're back frequently. Examine the brim/margin area of the hat with the cross. Check where the lid as well as the spore's surface is situated.

It's: Right is the point at which the time at the exact degree; no curved or lower curve: the edges of the depreciation arch. The head is bent and the cover is thin. lower arch of this.

Be involved: the credit card limit has been lowered.

Revolution: at the bottom of the hood curves upwards.

Rounded: Margin of payment.

Sterile: occurs when the lid's edge crosses the surface of the spore.

Take a look at the circuit's summary:

It's a smooth and full continuous contour. Casserole is characterized by its regular semicircles.

Striated ridges that are parallel and short.

Petals: The edges are cut backwards, just like areas of leaves.

Sinuados - Wavy edges.

Pekanie/Rimose: divided into the edges that surround the lid.

Appendix includes veins that form the border. Examine the texture and appearance on the inside of the hood. It's soft to skin.

Velvet: hair of a small size with delicately textured base.

Stairs: fibers that close and cover the lid, similar to stairs.

Wavy wrinkles in texture and appearance.

Hairy: Fibrous. It could be something that is dangerous.

Isolate: interrupted routine as painting. Warts: the traces of an old shop strewn across the upper floor. Wet and sticky (often located in the outdoors).

Wax: coating with an outer layer of smoothness.

Zone Colors: concentric groupings of color (e.g. turkey tail)

6. Determine the features of the antigen, or the surfaces of the spores. Take a look at the bottom of the sample, and then locate an area on the surface that is a spore. Be aware of your appearance. The most popular varieties are sheets, Gills on the floor, extremely small and fragile. Pores: decorative coating with pipesthat could be referred to as holes. Teeth are suspended icicle structures. False gills: ridges of meat that are hymen-related; they could resemble the gills (for instance or Chanterelles). Soil: meat in the shape of a ball which produces spores inside. Find the location where the gills meet connected to the stem and search to find a reason why they should be fixed. They are Free: the gills will not extend to the branch. Attached: the gills can be only located in the areas where the stem and the base meet. Decorative Attached to the stem to get all the length of the gill (right). The gills also pass through stem cells. Necklace: the gills can not connect to the stem cells however a chain joins them.

180

Sinuados: a strong record of gills before it slides a bit down the stem.

Examine the gills to determine the position of them beneath the lid. Are they overcrowded? The gills are closed: close up, making use of the space between them. Nearby The intestine is loose. The intestine is now in a good position. the gills.

7. Examine the stem and tree and evaluate the health for the trees. Check the lower portion of the stem, as well as the obstruction. It's central is located near the top of the cash register. Eccentric It is moved to the center on the cover. Side: handle aligned with entirety of the lid (not horizontal).

Sessile The answer is in no doubt about it. You must specify the stem type. Particularly, pay attention to the base which may be covered or underground.

It's equal in size of the trunk.

Fingernail: The stem grows gradually towards the bottom of the nail, much like pub.

Onion: the root of stem cells, often covered, could appear to be an onion.

Volva: a cup-shaped sachet on the base of the stem (remains of a veil that covers the entire globe).

Conical: The stem gets smaller at the lower. Radiation: A stem that is in a shaky root-shaped arrangement at the bottom.

Seek out the meaning or appearance. Check for color and other features. The stem's consistency is usually required for the development of porcini (stem cells, as well as the chickens protected jointly from the elements by porous pores).

Conclusion

I hope that you will enjoy reading this book. It was created so that the reader would be able to have a thorough understanding of the magic mushroom. Another reason for the book to be created was to help people know the advantages as well as the benefits of the magic mushroom, to ensure that they will be ready before using magic mushrooms.

If you have read the book,, you will be able to understand how people become dependent on magic mushrooms and how they can affect the human system.

www.ingramcontent.com/pod-product-compliance
Lightning Source LLC
Chambersburg PA
CBHW060333030426
42336CB00011B/1325